How to Eat Away ARTHRITIS

Lauri M. Aesoph, N.D.

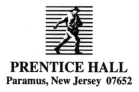

PRENTICE HALL
Paramus, New Jersey 07652

Library of Congress Cataloging-in-Publication Data

Aesoph, Lauri
   How to eat away arthritis / by Lauri Aesoph. — Rev. and expanded ed.
     p.   cm.
   Previously published under the title: How to eat away arthritis and gout /
  Norman D. Ford
   Includes index.
   ISBN 0-13-242900-4 (cloth). — ISBN 0-13-242892-X (pbk.)
    1. Arthritis—Diet therapy. 2. Gout—Diet therapy. 1. Ford, Norman
  D., 1921– How to eat away arthritis and gout. II. Title.
  RC933.F646 1996
  616.7'220654—dc20   96-23887
                                              CIP

Printed in the United States of America

10 9 8 7 6 5 4 3 (c)

10 9 8 7 6 5 4 3 (p)

This book is a reference work based on research by the author. The opinions expressed herein are nor necessarily those of or endorsed by the publisher. The suggestions and directions stated in the book are in no way to be considered as a substitute for consultation with a physician.

ISBN 0-13-242900-4 (c)

ISBN 0-13-242892-X (p)

ATTENTION: CORPORATIONS AND SCHOOLS

Prentice Hall books are available at quantity discounts with bulk purchase for educational, business, or sales promotional use. For information, please write to: Prentice Hall Career & Personal Development Special Sales, 240 Frisch Court, Paramus, New Jersey 07652. Please supply: title of book, ISBN number, quantity, how the book will be used, date needed.

PRENTICE HALL
Career & Personal Development
Paramus, NJ 07652
A Simon & Schuster Company

On the World Wide Web at http://www.phdirect.com

Prentice-Hall International (UK) Limited, *London*
Prentice-Hall of Australia Pty. Limited, *Sydney*
Prentice-Hall Canada Inc., *Toronto*
Prentice-Hall Hispanoamericana, S.A., *Mexico*
Prentice-Hall of India Private Limited, *New Delhi*
Prentice-Hall of Japan, Inc., *Tokyo*
Simon & Schuster Asia Pte. Ltd., *Singapore*
Editora Prentice-Hall do Brasil, Ltda., *Rio de Janeiro*

Contents

4. The Six Recovery Steps for Overcoming Arthritis 61

5. The Miracle Healing Technique That Banishes Most Arthritic Pain Within Seven Days 75

**9. Picking the Best Food Allergy Test for You—
    Including More Self-Help Methods 141**

Introduction

The food you eat can make your arthritis better or worse. This is not folklore or fiction—it is a scientific fact!

Using food as medicine is an ancient concept. For thousands of years healing traditions from around the world have relied on food to treat various conditions including arthritis. Today, scientists continue to uncover the medicinal and arthritic-fighting force of cayenne, fish, and other everyday foods. The foods have not changed, we just understand more.

Of course, battling arthritis is more than preparing select morsels; your diet must be full of health-building foods, too. In fact, using nutritious, wholesome foods to calm aching joints is a fundamental step still used by natural health practitioners everywhere to treat arthritis and gout. This book will teach you how to simply and inexpensively take this first nutritional step on your own.

If you want to stay on the road to recovery, you must also purge your meals of health-destroying foods—this idea has not changed. Removing these and other causes of arthritis, not merely masking symptoms with painkillers and other potentially harmful medicines, is the key to regaining robust health.

Caring for your entire body, not just swollen joints, is another vital part of treating arthritis. Did you know an ailing digestive tract can contribute to arthritic joints? Were you aware the immune system is tied to arthritis pain? Learning how this works and what to do about it is what natural medicine and this book are all about.

Many natural health experts shared specific therapies they use to treat arthritis patients for this revised edition. Also added are new scientific discoveries affirming the benefits of arthritis-eliminating foods. Read the still inspiring tales of men and women who have used nutrient-rich foods to repair and heal swollen joints . . . and more.

Are you surprised that, in this highly technological age, changing a basic habit like eating is such a powerful arthritis therapy? Don't be. Food and how we eat it forms the foundation of our well being.

This book will help anyone interested in improving their health. For the stories and information written here are not just about how diet can heal arthritis. On page after page, former arthritis victims and doctors reveal how vital, whole foods not only calm arthritis, but can unexpectedly relieve constipation, indigestion, and other chronic problems.

Nutrition is not the whole answer to treating arthritis, nor are bad eating habits the entire cause of this difficult disease. Long-time arthritis or even habitual use of certain medications may cause irreparable physical damage. But using our very basic, simple, and inexpensive up-to-date dietary suggestions can help improve or even eliminate your arthritic pain.

Happy reading and good eating.

Lauri M. Aesoph, ND

Chapter 1

How Restorative Foods Reverse Arthritis the Natural Way

You *can* eat away arthritis.

This is the message of the rapidly growing system of healing called natural medicine.

In fact alternative healing is becoming so popular that a 1990 survey estimated that one out of three Americans had used natural therapies in the past year to the tune of $13.7 billion [1].

Many conventional physicians consider a book suggesting that you can eat away arthritic disease scientifically unsound.

For years, the Arthritis Foundation has been warning Americans that arthritis is an incurable disease. The symptoms can be suppressed by drugs. But the disease is always there, ready to flare up again at any time. To make matters worse, the Arthritis Foundation warns us that "arthritis will be the epidemic of the future unless appropriate actions are taken now to limit its impact" [2].

According to the Foundation's rheumatologists—medical doctors specializing in arthritis—the cause of arthritic disease remains unclear—although theories continue to mount. Arthritic disease is a collective name for the hundred or so different varieties of arthritis, one of which is gout. According to the Foundation, no drug can permanently cure any one of these diseases.

The Arthritis Foundation admits that excess weight provokes osteoarthritis and includes food allergies, fasting, and fish oils as possible arthritis treatments[3]. However, it has flatly stated that with the possible exception of gout, no diet or food has any important beneficial or causative effect on arthritic disease[4].

But beginning in the late 1970s, a veritable explosion of new scientific information began to emerge from research institutions, medical centers and universities that first caused us to re-evaluate everything we previously knew and believed about arthritic disease. This research continues in full force today, and its ideas are seeping into conventional arthritic treatment.

A Modern Nutritional Miracle

From such widely varied branches of medicine as endocrinology, immunology, biochemistry, and nutrition, a mass of clinical evidence became available about previously unexplored areas of human nutrition. Although the answers are not all in yet, we already have at our disposal convincing proof that certain foods are a contributing cause of arthritic disease. More importantly, healthy joints seem dependent on gastrointestinal well-being.

Typical of the early research linking arthritis with a nutritional cause was the double-blind study conducted in 1979 by Dr. Anthony Conte, a Pittsburgh nutritionist, and his associate Dr. Marshall Mandell, a nationally-known allergist. According to reports, their study provided evidence that arthritis can be in many cases, an allergy-related disease that may be treated by simply avoiding certain common foods.

The study was conducted under rigorous scientific method using test subjects suffering from both rheumatoid and osteoarthritis—two main types of arthritic disease. Of these, 87 percent were found to have allergies that cause such typical arthritis symptoms as swelling and pain. The study results were presented to the American College of Allergists and published in the January 1980 issue of *Annals of Allergy*.

In the following weeks and months, identical reports that arthritis is a nutrition caused disease began to filter in from physicians and scientists who were conducting similar but separate studies of their own.

For example, Dr. Robert Stroud, a prominent rheumatologist at the University of Alabama School of Medicine, is reportedly one of many scientists to have done pioneering work to show that patients with arthritic disease respond very favorably when certain foods are eliminated from their diet.

Even more dramatic is the fact that for many people, arthritis symptoms completely clear up during a fast. This proves that food plays an important role in the development and treatment of arthritis. However, you can't fast forever.

Fortunately, scientists have expanded on the food allergy theory during the past decade. Drs. L. G. Darlington and N. W. Ramsey, British rheumatologists from Epsom General Hospital, wrote a letter to *The Lancet*, a respected English medical journal, describing their successes using diet to treat rheumatoid arthritis. One-third of their 100 patients were still well after seven and a half years of diet-only treatment (that's not to say that diet didn't help others). Besides food intolerance, the doctors said the foods you eat can influence your digestive tract, the bacteria in your gut and inflammation—all which ultimately affect arthritis [5].

 ## Nutritional Science Has Already Unlocked Some Secrets to Arthritic Disease

As we stand on the threshold of this exciting new knowledge, it is becoming increasingly clear that arthritis is not the incurable diseases we once believed.

What these doctors and scientists are now saying is that many forms of arthritis are aggravated by foods. While food allergies don't cause arthritis, they may, along with poor eating habits and genetic susceptibility, encourage your body to attack its own joints.

For further confirmation that arthritis is a food-linked disease, consider the results of recent studies drawing a connection between what scientists called the "leaky gut syndrome" and autoimmune disorders, like rheumatoid arthritis. Some arthritic individuals have sieve-like gastrointestinal tracts that allow partially digested food and other substances to seep into their bloodstream. This is how food allergies and possibly allergy to your own body, called autoimmunity, happens.

Thus medical science has at last confirmed what old-time folk healers have said for years—that certain health destroying foods are a primary reason for arthritis. By replacing them with certain health restoring foods, we definitely can encourage remission of this disease together with elimination of stiffness, pain, and inflammation.

Nutritional Therapy Has Outdated Medical Treatment

These important new advances have outdated orthodox medicine's capability to treat arthritis. We now have available a mass of new data linking arthritic disease with nutrition that simply did not exist when several present doctors were attending medical school.

But instead of welcoming these discoveries, as you might expect, conventional medical practitioners have almost totally ignored them. For most doctors and rheumatologists are too busy, overworked, and locked-in by their own medical school training to keep abreast of new discoveries.

Arthur H. Discovers That Drugs Are Not the Only Way to Get Well

Take the case of Arthur H. whose doctor had been treating him for rheumatoid arthritis for seven years. Arthur finally became so frustrated with his doctor's lack of success that he consulted an allergist. Sensitivity tests revealed that Arthur had developed allergic responses to milk, wheat, and potatoes. When Arthur eliminated these foods from his diet, the arthritis disappeared within two weeks.

Arthur returned to his original doctor to tell about his success, but the doctor was unimpressed. He made no attempt to seek information about nutritional therapy from the allergist. Nor did he refer any of his arthritic patients there. Instead he simply went on prescribing drugs just as he had been taught in medical school.

Medical Science Is Gradually Turning Around

Past experience has shown that the lag time between the discovery of an important therapy and the time that doctors actually accept and use it is often as much as 20 or 30 years. For example, it took almost 30 years from the time that diet and exercise therapy were demonstrated to be able to reverse heart disease until cardiac rehabilitation centers began to appear.

It's been nearly 15 years since we first brought you this news. So hopefully your doctor is using some nutritional therapy to treat arthritis. If not, point him in the direction of the numerous published studies on the subject. Still, most doctors will continue to say that you must learn to live with your arthritis. And they will continue to prescribe noxious drugs as the main answer to inflammation and pain.

Revolution in Nutrition Reveals Cause of Arthritis

How can this plethora of new scientific findings help you reverse arthritis?

For at least 150 years (in some healing traditions, millennia), we've known that arthritic disease could be benefited and often permanently reversed by changing to a diet of fresh, natural, health-restoring foods. The disease usually disappeared for as long as the person stayed on the diet.

But not everyone was able to recover fully by changing their diet. Recent scientific discoveries have now revealed why.

Arthritis is not, as was previously thought, caused simply by eating devitalized, health robbing foods. Nutritional research has now discovered that food influences arthritic disease in two distinct stages. In the first stage, the nutritional deficiency caused by eating depleted, processed foods paves the way for a second stage consisting of one or more food allergies. It is these allergic reactions that may trigger our immune system to attack the tissue in our joints.

This explains why, in past times, some people who made a complete changeover from health destroying foods to health-restoring foods never completely got rid of arthritis. They still had allergies to one or more of the natural foods. We are also learning the tremendous importance of healing the gut and improving overall health.

We now have so much important new knowledge concerning arthritis that we are witnessing a whole series of modern nutritional miracles.

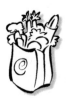

Be Your Own Nutritional Therapist

Among them is the discovery that you yourself can easily test and identify the exact culprit foods that are creating the allergy that may be causing your arthritis. You can use some of the identical tests that a professional allergist would make, and you can do it all easily and simply in the privacy of your own home without experience, equipment, or expense.

Other important discoveries show that the way you eat also affects the way you feel. Having a strongly positive attitude can halve the time it takes to recover from arthritis. Eat right and you'll feel right.

But what really swings the odds in your favor is the discovery that the more you know about arthritis the more power it gives you over the disease.

The purpose of this book is to show how you can use this totally natural nutritional approach to lessen or even relieve the pain and inflammation of arthritis and to restore yourself to perfect health.

Restorative Foods—The Natural Approach to Healing Arthritis

New knowledge has come from the research frontiers of psychology and behavioral motivation to show that when you change your diet, you simultaneously benefit your whole person on the physical, mental, and emotional levels.

Natural medicine, once the property of folk healers and fringe practitioners, is quickly gaining respect in this country. While natural health healers range from scientifically trained naturopathic physicians and chiropractors to self-taught herbalists, the principles of natural medicine remain the same.

The natural approach to health says that total health is possible only when the whole person is functioning smoothly. The natural approach is not merely to ease pain and swelling but to end arthritic disease altogether by *removing the cause.*

The natural approach to arthritis says that drugs are not the only option. Nutrition is one of several gentle, alternative therapies that have proven as equally—sometimes more—effective than conventional care.

As a result, the natural rationale is creating a revolution in our approach to disease. Simply because conventional medical treatment is the established way to treat an ailment, it is not necessarily the only way.

The reason is, of course, that arthritis is made worse by our own incorrect eating habits. It has also been amply demonstrated that our health destroying foods are largely the cause of a whole class of degenerative diseases that includes heart disease, stroke, atherosclerosis, hypertension, adult-onset diabetes, diverticulosis, and chronic headaches.

What arthritis and all these diseases have in common is that they are not caused by a virus or a bacterium that could be wiped out by drugs. They are often activated instead by our life-wrecking eating habits.

To say diet causes all disease is too simplistic. Fallen health is the result of a chain of events beginning with genetics and fostered by stress overload, a sedentary existence, and pollution. However, the foods we eat and how we eat them can swing the health pendulum from well to sick. Cultures that still eat a primitive diet chock full of unprocessed, whole foods rarely contract civilized disease like arthritis. Easy living and poor eating has made us sicker. One way to reverse these diseases is to eliminate the cause, that is, by rehabilitating our suicidal eating habits.

Drugs cannot alter what we eat. Hence it should come as no surprise that mainstream medicine has yet to produce a single bonafide cure for any of the degenerative diseases.

All that medical science can do is to mask or suppress or cut out the symptoms of these diseases. Aspirin may temporarily alleviate the pain and swelling of rheumatoid arthritis, but neither aspirin nor any other drugs can cure arthritic disease. In fact, aspirin and other pain killers may even accelerate joint damage in diseases like osteoarthritis[6]. On the other hand, a natural therapy like nutrition can only help.

A Simple Diet Change Ends Both Arthritis and Migraine for Betty M.

Ever since she was 18, Betty M. had suffered from frequent migraine headaches. At age 31, after the birth of her second child, Betty began to experience stiffness and pain in her left knee on rising. Soon the pain and swelling spread to her fingers, wrists, and ankles. Based on lab tests, her doctor diagnosed rheumatoid arthritis.

Within 18 months, Betty was so wracked by agonizing joint pains that she was unable to walk or do housework. Meanwhile her headaches became even more excruciating. Altogether her doctor prescribed 16 aspirin daily with Nalfon and Tolectin plus routine shots of cortisone. But nothing helped. Her doctor admitted that the drugs could only suppress symptoms. He told Betty that the cause of rheumatoid arthritis was unknown and the disease was medically incurable.

One day, Betty read about the benefits of natural foods in a health magazine. Out of sheer frustration she decided to act. She hobbled downstairs and dragged out every canned, packaged, and convenience food in the house. When her husband came home, she had him replace them with natural health restoring foods just as the magazine had recommended.

Ten days later, the pain and swelling in her joints began to subside. And simultaneously her migraine headaches began to taper off.

In six weeks time, Betty was well enough to walk and resume housework and her headaches had also disappeared. A naturopathic physician whom she consulted explained her recovery as due to the fact that both the arthritis and migraine had been caused by the devitalized foods on which she had lived for years. When the cause—the health-destroying foods—was removed, both diseases disappeared.

We can't guarantee anything, of course. But if you already have another degenerative disease (cancer excepted) in addition to arthritis, you may notice an improvement in the other disease as well as in the arthritic disease. For all degenerative diseases are aggravated by our same incorrect lifestyle habits. When we remove this irritant by cleaning up our habits, chances are good that any of these other diseases you have may also gradually disappear.

 ## Drugs Treat Symptoms of Arthritis, Not the Cause

As researchers and scientists assess this new information, many have already reached a rather obvious but nonetheless startling conclusion.

Arthritis, along with most other degenerative diseases, *are simply not curable by medication*. Our medical schools have not trained doctors to recognize the cause of degenerative diseases nor to treat them by therapies that actually work.

Even cutting out a diseased organ does not remove the cause. When a heart patient with cholesterol choked coronary arteries is given new arteries in a by-pass operation, absolutely nothing is accomplished towards removing the cause of his disease.

Often, within as short a time as one year, the new arteries again become choked with cholesterol caused by the same high-fat diet which blocked the original arteries. The only "cure" for heart disease that really works is to change to a diet of health restoring foods.

So even heart disease is not really a problem solved with surgery and drugs. As with arthritis, the "cure" lies in something we can do for ourselves. That "something" is to use nutritional therapy to change our life-threatening eating habits. We can become our own nutritional therapists. Instead of cutting out organs, we can cut out at least one cause of arthritic disease.

Because conventional medical science has no bonafide cure for any degenerative disease, natural oriented healers prefer to avoid using the word "cure." Instead, they talk about "reversing" gout or arthritis. Many degenerative diseases can be reversed and kept in a state of remission only as long as a person practices healthful living habits. Even infectious diseases, usually "cured" with a germ-killing drug, can be avoided with proper eating and healthful living.

When gout sufferer John R. changed to a diet of low-fat natural foods, his gout soon disappeared. For 3 years John stayed strictly with his diet without a further trace of gout. Then he became careless and while on a cruise ate several meals of rich meats with wine. A few days later he hobbled off the ship with both big toes swollen, hot, tender, and throbbing.

Strategy for Recovery

This book is not written to challenge conventional medical treatment. We most strongly urge and recommend anyone with any kind of chronic or persistent pain to consult a physician for a professional diagnosis.

Arthritis-like pains, such as stiffness, swelling, and inflammation of one or more joints can be caused by a variety of infectious diseases. Hepatitis, strep and staph infections, TB, pneumonia, meningitis, syphilis, and gonorrhea can all create symptoms similar to those of arthritis. Untreated cases of advanced gout have also caused hypertension, renal disease, diabetes, and heart disease.

These diseases may be medical emergencies which, if not treated, can cause rapid and permanent destruction to joints, heart, kidneys, eyes, and other vital organs. When these diseases are cured with antibiotics or other emergency treatment, the arthritic symptoms quickly disappear. Using emergency treatment to cure infections and other diseases of rapid onset has been conventional medicine's greatest triumph.

That's not to say that natural medicine can't help these conditions. A professional trained in natural therapeutics can tell you if alternative treatments are appropriate for what ails you. It's also very fitting to use natural remedies as an adjunct to drugs and surgery, to both speed healing and decrease side effects. The trouble is that conventional medicine uses the same kind of emergency treatment to deal with degenerative diseases that often take years to appear.

No Cure for Arthritis in the Medicine Bottle

Although conventional medicine is opening its eyes to the benefits of exercise and other lifestyle changes, treatment for arthritis invariably begins with drugs. For example, as many as 16 or more aspirin per day may be prescribed to relieve pain and inflammation, a treatment you must continue daily for life. When aspirin doesn't work, or worse yet, makes you sicker, another drug—usually one of the NSAID (non-steroidal anti-inflammatory drug) family like ibuprofen or acetaminophen—is prescribed.

While nutritional science is gaining favor among rheumatologists, most arthritis research in the last 15 years has focused on new and better drugs. The NSAID list (which includes aspirin and other salicylates as a subset) now totals 20 or more different kinds[7]. Over two billion dollars worth of NSAID drugs were sold in 1994 alone[8].

Aspirin, the "jack of all trades" when it comes to pain, and its NSAID cousins reduce pain and inflammation by blocking the production of hormone-like compounds called prostaglandins. These substances are usually made by your body's immune system to defend itself against infection and to promote healing by initiating the swelling, heat, stiffness, tenderness, and redness of inflammation. However, in the case of rheumatoid arthritis, the immune system is out of control and prostaglandins are churned out at an incredible rate. The result is red swollen joints.

Even though aspirin and NSAIDs soothe symptoms and curtail prostaglandin production, it's a quick fix. Reining in prostaglandins isn't such a bad idea—naturopathic physicians do this all the time for various inflammatory conditions including arthritis. But if you only reduce prostaglandins and don't pay attention to the nutritional causes of arthritis, you're right back where you started.

The harsher drug cure is hard on the patient—you. Read this quote from the *Textbook of Rheumatology*, a mainstream medical textbook:

> As every practicing physician quickly learns, the more aggressive and potent is the pharmacologic attempt nonspecifically to suppress this reaction (inflammation), the more defenseless the resulting host. The preoccupation of rheumatologists with nonspecific anti-inflammatory remedies reflects our ignorance of the specific proximate or ultimate causes of many of the diseases we are called upon to treat[9].

In other words, doctors use anti-inflammatory drugs because they don't know what causes arthritis. And these medicines ruin your ability to fight illness. Drugs' side effects are a problem too.

In an *Arthritis Today* article entitled "Following Doctor's Order's . . ." Christopher Lorish, PhD, assistant professor of physical therapy at the University of Alabama at Birmingham School of Health Related Professions, says drug side effects are the most common reason patients give for refusing or skipping medications[10].

In its booklet *Arthritis The Basic Facts*, the Arthritis Foundation admits that aspirin taken in large doses can cause stomach irritation and ringing in the ears.

But according to the British medical journal *Lancet*, when cardiac patients took three or more aspirin a day on a long-term basis, ten-to-twenty percent experienced dyspepsia, nausea, and vomiting.

A report by Walter W. Ross in the December 1980 issue of *Reader's Digest* (page 133) states that of every 100,000 persons who seek medical attention for severe gastro intestinal bleeding, ten-to-fifteen percent have this condition as a result of regular aspirin use. A 1988 British study found that aspirin and other NSAIDs accounted for more than one-third of bleeding peptic ulcers in people over 60[11]. In the U.S. NSAID-associated gastric ulcers are estimated to cost more than $100 million per year[12]. As a matter of course many doctors prescribe, along with pain pills, anti-ulcer medicines to both prevent and treat aspirin or NSAID-induced ulcers[7].

Everyone who takes aspirin loses approximately half a teaspoon of blood from the stomach lining with each tablet taken. Regular aspirin use can lead to asthma, skin eruptions, kidney malfunction, colon ulceration, and problems in vision and taste.

Ross' report concludes that if aspirin were to be discovered today and tested by modern standards, it would be obtainable only by prescription.

The NSAIDs acetominophen (Tylenol™) and ibuprofen have become almost as prevalent as aspirin for arthritis pain. Unfortunately, these increasingly popular drugs merely have different side effects (in some cases more serious than aspirin). For example, besides causing stomach problems, some NSAIDs can hurt your liver[13].

Judith P. Wishes She'd Picked Naturopathy Not Drugs

Judith P. from Watertown, Massachusetts, shared her frustrations regarding drug therapy in a letter to *Arthritis Today* (January/February 1996), a magazine for arthritis sufferers published by the Arthritis Foundation. She expressed her frustration about the huge profits made by drug companies, adding "(it) seems the Arthritis Foundation subscribes fully to such (drug-base) approaches to disease treatment."

When a doctor was quoted in the magazine as saying "because there are effective drugs that have been tested for the management of arthritis available to you, there is no need for homeopathic medicine," Ms. Poole responded with: "This ignores the fact that anti-inflammatory drugs are known to have potent side effects. Tolerance for them varies. I suffered with an ulcer and now have compromised kidney function from the use of NSAIDs. I wish that I had turned to naturopathic and homeopathic treatment sooner"[14].

The Grim Side Effects of Arthritis Drugs

When these fail, treatment moves on to steroids, powerful anti-inflammatory drugs but with such adverse side effects they can be used only in very low doses for very short periods. Still, steroids like prednisone are used for 10 or more years by some people with rheumatoid arthritis. Dr. John Sibley, a Canadian rheumatologist from the Royal University Hospital in Saskatoon, Saskatchewan, found patients who used prednisone for a decade did poorly. Not only was their arthritis worse than their steroid-free counterparts, but fractures and cataracts were more of a problem[15]. Gold salts are another drug treatment with extremely limited use because of devastating side effects. "Many doctors fear the unknown," was the opinion of an editorial in The Lancet, "and will settle for an old friend even if there is associated toxicity. Perhaps this is why gold (an expensive, dangerous, and often ineffective drug) still has so many proponents"[16].

Among other medical treatments are anti-malarial drugs which are also notorious for severe side effects. And among the more experimental drugs are cytotoxic agents, identical to those used in transplant operations to suppress the immune system. Hair loss and intestinal upsets are common among users.

To some extent, cytotoxic drugs and gold do relieve rheumatoid arthritis by inhibiting the immune system. Interestingly enough, they do so by suppressing the white blood cell population, the very same cells that have been found to multiply in response to food allergies. These surplus cells then attack joint tissue, thus causing rheumatoid and similar varieties of arthritis.

Through using cytotoxic agents on human guinea pigs, conventional medical science has helped prove that food allergies are, indeed, one contributing cause of rheumatoid arthritis.

 ## Nutrient Downslide with Drugs

It's not enough that drugs may have harmful, and at the very least, uncomfortable side effects. Many arthritis medicines also rob you of valuable vitamins and minerals. Think about this for a minute.

Not only are eating habits central to healing arthritis, but medications prescribed by your doctor to treat this disease make mediocre eating habits even worse. Aspirin, a nutritional time bomb, steals iron, folic acid, and vitamins C, B1, and K from you[17]. (See Appendix B for "Drugs that Steal Nutrients"). We only need small amounts of these and other nutrients for survival, but without them we become very sick or die.

Vitamins and minerals play a number of roles in the body ranging from metabolism to converting food into energy. Scientists are also discovering how important specific nutrients are for optimal immunity.

Modern society is fraught with nutritional bandits. Stress from noise, pollution, overcrowding, and other daily demands misappropriate vitamins and minerals. Today's soil is suffering from its own nutrient deficiencies due to modern farming practices. Processing and refining strip whole foods. If this weren't enough, storing and cooking foods withdraw more nutritional value. Older individuals— the group hardest hit by arthritis—has its own set of special nutritional needs.

If you add nutrient robbing drugs to an already taxed diet, you begin to understand why standard American fare hardly, if ever, meets daily nutritional requirements. The higher nutritional demands of arthritic disease are certainly out of reach.

Drugs—The Arthritis Remedy That Makes You Sicker

As of this writing, we can say that not a single one of these drugs can cure arthritis. A review of their various side effects includes such conditions as nausea, vomiting, headaches, impotence, hypertension, severe bone loss, confusion, drowsiness, insomnia, double vision, moon face, and deep personality changes. Many arthritis drugs have already fallen into disrepute due to their excessive and intolerable side effects. To cap it all, the drugs often fail to relieve either pain or inflammation. Some even promote joint degeneration.

In reality, not a single drug in the entire pharmacopoeia is entirely free of side effects. Every single drug shows a toxic allergy response in food tolerance tests.

All of which means that drugs actually intensify and worsen overall health, immunity and the very arthritic diseases which they are supposed to relieve.

Medicine's No-Win Pessimism Can Be More Crippling Than Arthritis Itself

If all this conflicting advice by doctors sounds confusing, it is. On one hand, we have doctors of conventional medicine telling us that arthritic disease is medically incurable and can be treated mainly with drugs. On the other, in total contradiction, a new breed of naturally oriented M.D.s and naturopathic physicians are telling us that arthritis can be reversed with nutritional and other natural therapies.

These alternative physicians are also highly critical of the discouraging no-win advice given to arthritis sufferers by the Arthritis Foundation and the allopathic medical profession. Numerous medical studies have already proved the value of the placebo effect. Because arthritis is presumed incurable by some doctors doesn't mean it cannot be reversed or improved by other safe and effective approaches.

In its booklet *Arthritis The Basic Facts*, the Foundation states: ". . . the major forms of arthritis are chronic. This means the condition, once started, continues, usually for life. It means that one does not 'heal up as good as new' as after a common cold, measles, or a cut in the skin. It means that whatever damage takes place may remain permanently . . . and tend to get worse unless proper precautions are taken to prevent it. It means that treatment must continue on and on."

The same booklet has these discouraging words to say about gout: "Medications to keep uric acid levels down must be continued for life. Medication controls rather than cures the disease."

Doctors in Conflict

Today, thousands of health professionals trained in natural medicine believe that this negative advice destroys all incentive to try to recover through an alternative therapy. The pessimistic prognosis given by most doctors crushes all expectations of recovery and any hope that joints will move freely once more.

Such a gloomy view closes the door to any therapy but drugs. It destroys all hope, faith, and belief that health can be restored. And it effectively discourages anyone from taking an active role in his or her own recovery.

It is not our intent to raise false hopes, but part of the emerging knowledge about arthritis concerns the tremendous power that suggestion plays in boosting recovery. Studies have shown that people with strongly positive attitudes who firmly believe they will get well can expect to recover from any disease or injury in 25–50 percent less time than someone with a negative, passive, and helpless attitude.

In contrast, the power of orthodox medicine's negative suggestions can be more crippling then the disease itself.

Health-Building Foods Work Naturally to Give Mary R. a Positive, Get-Well Attitude

The decision to change your diet is the turning point in recovery from arthritis. The moment you decide to stop being a passive recipient of drugs and to strike out and act on your own, you subconsciously transform yourself from a helpless, disease-prone individual into a cheerful, positive, optimistic person in full control of your own body, mind, and destiny.

At 42, Mary R. was a typical rheumatoid arthritis sufferer who had developed a deep sense of helplessness through being told by her doctor that cure was impossible and that she must learn to live with arthritis for the rest of her life. Her attitude became increasingly dependent and passive.

By the end of her second year with the disease, Mary had mentally turned her body over to her doctor. "Drug me. Cut me open. Make me well," were her thoughts each time she saw her doctor. Mary believed that her health was beyond her control and she mentally transferred all responsibility to her physician.

One day, Mary heard an evangelist on the radio who urged listeners to wake up and take charge of their lives and their health. She felt suddenly inspired. She tossed out her aspirins and abruptly dropped from taking 14 a day to taking none (a course not advised in this book).

At the same time she consulted a chiropractor who specialized in nutrition. She was advised to immediately change to a diet of fresh, natural foods and to stay strictly away from all processed, canned, and convenience foods.

That night, Mary suffered the worst flare-up she had ever experienced. Without analgesics to ease the pain, the agony was torturous. But she grimly held on. By the end of the second day the continuous pain had subsided. Slowly, the heat and swelling in her joints gradually improved.

That was four years ago. Only once, immediately following a nutritional lapse, has Mary experienced a flare-up. But she returned immediately to her diet and has had no more pain. Today, she swims, hikes, and practices yoga. Arthritis is just a memory.

Her chiropractor, a firm believer in the natural approach, told Mary that alternative medicine does not accept as final the stereo-typed assumption shared by most doctors that adults are not willing to change their lifestyle habits.

As he told Mary: "The natural approach is that if you *sincerely* desire to be free of pain, you will take an active role in your own recovery."

Only You Can Heal Yourself

Treating arthritis yourself by nutritional therapy is not as easy as popping a pill. It demands that you become actively involved in your own recovery by making permanent changes in your eating habits.

The reason is that the body is a self-healing entity that will heal itself *when the cause of disease is removed.*

Once we remove the cause of arthritis by eliminating sickness-breeding foods, the body's own recuperative powers will go to work to restore health.

Other important discoveries show that the way you eat also affects the way you feel. Gulping down food while rushing from place to place just creates indigestion. And as you'll soon learn, good digestion is crucial to mending arthritic joints.

Identifying foods that aggravate your arthritis is also important on the road to wellness. While you can identify food intolerances on your own, you may prefer having your doctor perform a simple blood test to detect food culprits. Later on, we'll point out the pros and cons of each method.

But what really swings the odds in your favor is realizing that the more you know about arthritis, the more power it gives you over the disease.

The body is you. It is not something you can turn over to a doc-tor and expect him to make you well. Drugs cannot remove the wrong habits that are the cause of arthritis. Only you can heal arthritic dis-ease. No one else can do it for you.

Marjorie W.'s Arthritis Pains Vanish in Six Days When She Becomes Her Own Nutritional Therapist

For ten years, Marjorie W. had suffered increasing pains from rheumatoid arthritis. Life became a continual horror of drugs, pain, and sleepless nights. Nothing seemed to help. Finally, Marjorie's hands became so stiff and swollen that she underwent an operation by a specialist.

For five weeks following the operation, Marjorie was unable to use her hands at all. Then her fingers became even stiffer than before.

During her ten years with arthritis, Marjorie's doctors had prescribed a total of 15 different medications ranging from aspirin to steroids and powerful narcotics. But all they produced was distressing side effects. Finally, Marjorie could no longer comb her hair. After years of suffering, she became resigned to being physically impaired for life.

Throughout her years of torment, Marjorie had always assumed that arthritis was something over which she had no control. Healing was something that could come only from a doctor's prescription.

Quite by accident, she learned about natural healing and the benefits of nutritional therapy. Out of sheer desperation she decided to give it a try.

Marjorie enrolled at Villa Vegetariana, a nutritional health school in Mexico. The doctor in charge was appalled by the long list of health-wrecking foods that Marjorie ate each day. Her own doctor had never mentioned a word about diet. Marjorie was immediately placed on a natural self-purification technique designed to detoxify her whole body.

Exactly six days after she stopped eating her usual foods, Marjorie was astounded to find herself completely free of pain. At this point, she was placed on a diet of fresh fruits and vegetables. Eight days later, full use of her hands returned.

Each evening, Marjorie attended a lecture to learn how she was to eat for the rest of her life. She was advised to adopt a lifetime diet of fresh, natural, high-fiber foods.

Although she was then 62, an age at which most doctors believe our habits have become totally inflexible, Marjorie found no difficulty in adapting to her new way of eating.

For several years now she has stayed strictly with her diet of health-restoring foods. Not a single flare-up has occurred. And she has felt absolutely no urge to return to her former eating habits.

Marjorie no longer views natural foods as a hardship. She leads a completely normal, active life and she regards giving up trouble-making foods as a small price to pay for total freedom from arthritis.

Although she didn't realize it at the time, Marjorie's decision to act by changing her diet was the turning point in her recovery. Her decision to become actively involved expressed a powerful belief in her own body's ability to get well.

Are you ready to do the same?

Chapter *2*

The Wonder Working Power of Restorative Foods

This book began when Norman Ford, a writer in retirement, developed an interest in arthritis. Each year for 30 years he talked with hundreds of men and women in adult communities throughout the Sunbelt States. When Ford originally did his research, approximately one retirement-aged American in four suffered pain and discomfort from some form of arthritis. Today nearly half of all Americans over 65 are so affected[18]. Since arthritic disease is a major deterrent to enjoyment of the later years, he made a point of finding out everything he could about arthritis and the chances for recovery.

Judging by the many people he met who were crippled by the agonizing pain of rheumatoid arthritis—a common form of arthritic disease—arthritis did indeed seem to be as incurable as the Arthritis Foundation claimed. As their booklet *Arthritis The Basic Facts* states: "The cause of rheumatoid arthritis is not yet known. A cure is not yet known. . . . No drug yet developed for use in treating rheumatoid arthritis actually stops the basic disease process."

If by the Arthritis Foundation's own admission, the major forms of arthritis are incurable, and cannot be stopped by drugs, then why, Ford wondered, *did I keep meeting people who claimed to have experienced a complete and permanent remission from rheumatoid and other forms of arthritis?*

Fifteen years later, Dr. Lauri Aesoph was asked to update this information. After purusing the scientific literature and talking with several doctors specializing in natural health, she discovered that the original author's observations about food and arthritis was even truer today.

As part of his arthritis-inquiry program, Ford made regular visits to some of the small Nature Cure resorts and natural diet arthritis clinics that dot Florida and the Southwest. And he began to attend natural food conventions. At these places, Ford met more men and women—people in all age brackets—who had achieved total and lasting remission from all forms of arthritis and gout. One of them was Enid C.

Enid C. Gets Out of Her Wheelchair and Walks

Three years after she had been stricken with rheumatoid arthritis, 41-year-old Enid C.'s knees were so swollen she had to give up her teaching job and take to a wheelchair. Enid's doctor tried all the usual drugs but without success. Finally, in desperation, Enid consulted a practitioner of natural hygiene (a science of natural health).

The hygienist instructed Enid to practice a simple self-purification technique for seven days, then to eat light, nutritious meals of fresh natural foods. She was to stay on this diet permanently.

On the evening of the seventh day of the purification technique, Enid suddenly realized that her arthritis pains had vanished. Two weeks later, the swelling in her knees had almost disappeared.

Exactly six weeks after she first visited the hygienist, Enid got out of her wheelchair and walked—entirely free of stiffness and pain. In another three months she was back teaching school.

Enid has stayed faithfully with her restorative foods and has been completely free of arthritis symptoms for over three years.

21,000 Americans Recover Annually from "Incurable" Rheumatoid Arthritis

According to the Arthritis Foundation, a remission, ". . . is the medical word used when a disease seems to go away by itself. The pain, stiffness, and swelling of arthritis, even in severe cases, may subside or disappear for months or years. *In about one out of ten cases it never comes back.*"

The italics are ours. But here, based on government surveys of tens of thousands of arthritis patients, is the official word. IN ABOUT ONE OUT OF TEN CASES RHEUMATOID ARTHRITIS SPONTANEOUSLY DISAPPEARS AND NEVER COMES BACK.

Since 2,100,000[18] Americans suffer from rheumatoid arthritis at any one time, this means that approximately 21,000 people achieve a permanent and complete remission from rheumatoid arthritis every year—whether or not they receive medical treatment.

Of all the people Ford talked with who had, or had previously suffered from, rheumatoid arthritis, approximately one in ten reported that, like Enid C., they had experienced a full and lasting remission. This seemed to agree entirely with the Foundation's own estimate that in about one out of ten cases rheumatoid arthritis never comes back.

Arthritis Recovery Secret Revealed

What was their secret? Why, Ford wondered, did one person out of ten with rheumatoid arthritis recover completely with or without standard medical care?

Starting about 30 years ago, each time Ford met a person who had recovered from any form of arthritic disease, he tried to find out what was different about him or her compared to others who still had the disease.

Almost every person he questioned had run the whole gamut of conventional medical treatment, usually without any significant relief or improvement.

Yet out of their answers a common pattern gradually emerged. In virtually every case, recovery occurred when, by accident or design, each person had decided to give his body a chance to heal itself. With few exceptions, each person Ford questioned had made a radical improvement in living habits just prior to recovery.

 ## Astonishing Benefits from a Change in Diet

Some had cut out smoking or alcohol. But far more reported having made a major change in their eating habits, usually by switching to a diet of fresh, natural, unprocessed foods.

Surprisingly, the majority had not done so in the belief that they could reverse their arthritis but in response to the numerous books and articles urging Americans to reduce their risk of heart disease by losing weight and eating less fat. For some 30 years we have been repeatedly told that a natural diet of high-fiber foods reduces risk of heart disease, diabetes, hypertension, diverticulosis, and other degenerative diseases.

Americans were not told that it would also improve arthritis. But, in practice, a surprising number of former arthritis sufferers seem to have benefited.

In more recent years more men and women are changing their diets by enrolling at cardiac rehabilitation centers. Actual records from cardiac centers show that the same low-fat, high-fiber diet of natural foods that helps reverse heart disease may also benefit arthritis.

A smaller number of people had deliberately changed their diet through reading that natural foods could benefit arthritic disease. Others had learned about nutritional therapy from friends, nutritionists, and chiropractors. A few like Marjorie W., (see Chapter 1) had enrolled at one of the small natural health resorts scattered about the country where they had rehabilitated their diet under the guidance of nutritionists.

One way or another, by luck or coincidence, these people had learned about the benefits of nutritional therapy and had decided to take the initiative and give it a try.

Why There Is No Anti-Arthritis Diet for Everyone

Not all of the people who had changed their diets had successfully recovered from arthritic disease. Although all felt greatly improved, approximately four in ten had failed to recover completely.

A few years ago it was not known why this was so.

Yet today we know there is no such thing as an anti-arthritic diet that will work for everyone. The information avalanche of recent years has revealed that while some foods are so devitalized they inevitably lead everyone towards poorer health, including arthritic disease for some, each of us may also have our own individual allergies to specific arthritis-aggravating foods.

This is one reason why in past times a changeover to a natural diet benefited many arthritis sufferers but not all. Several who were not able to improve their arthritis significantly had allergies that extended even to some natural foods.

Due to the new work on arthritis therapy, the foods that aggravate some forms of arthritic disease can be identified by you.

This is not to deny the tremendous therapeutic value of natural foods in reversing both arthritic and other degenerative diseases. In heart disease, hypertension, maturity-onset diabetes, osteoporosis, obesity, senility, diverticulosis, hypoglycemia, colitis, and similar diseases brought on by the vicissitudes of our own lifestyles, the best place to start is with a diet of natural foods.

But some types of arthritis differ in that they are also autoimmune diseases. This means that the nutritional deficiencies caused by eating devitalized, processed foods disturb digestion and may pave the way for food allergies that can trigger white blood cells to attack the cells in our joints.

Thus a complete remission often requires digestive healing and the elimination of specific allergy foods.

 ## Recovery Program Combines Nature's Secrets with Modern Nutritional Science

Many of Ford's observations fit together with the latest discoveries of nutritional science like a jigsaw puzzle.

Scientific information then and now explained why all of the scores of people interviewed had been able to improve or recover from arthritis.

This book synthesizes all the scattered, pigeonholed discoveries of hundreds of people who have recovered from arthritis with the findings of scores of doctors and researchers, and meshes it into a collection of nutritional therapy successfully employed to reverse arthritis by natural health establishments.

When put all together, what emerges is a simple, workable program consisting of Six Recovery Steps that anyone can use to greatly benefit their arthritis.

We want to emphasize that the Six Recovery Steps are not "our" program. And this information is not meant to replace the services of your doctor or a skilled natural health practitioner.

All we have actually done is to integrate the methods used to improve arthritis by the hundreds of people interviewed with the most successful natural therapies currently being used by the many small allergy and arthritis clinics and natural healing centers across the country.

So while the Six Recovery Steps program is not based entirely on recent discoveries, the methods used *have* been proven successful by the well authenticated and scientifically validated work of many university scientists and research physicians.

Chapter by chapter, the case histories collected over the years provide living proof of the effectiveness of each of the Six Recovery Steps.

What You Should Expect from the Six Recovery Steps

The program described is based on medically sound methods that are already being used with great success in a number of small allergy and arthritis clinics. Some are experimental units associated with major universities and medical research centers. Several respected natural health doctors are also using these methods.

Changing the way you eat is the focus of this arthritis self-help book. And truthfully, every health program (and disease treatment) should always start with a nutritional overhaul. Such a basic concept is overlooked by too many doctors. However, there's more to arthritis and other degenerative diseases than diet.

While revising this book, we spoke to many natural health doctors who all agreed that nutrition was basic to healing arthritis, but eating poorly doesn't create swollen joints in everyone. Genetic susceptibility, your body's weak point, needs to be considered. So while eating processed foods might aggravate your rheumatoid arthritis, it could cause heart disease in someone else.

Other factors besides diet have to be considered too. There's no doubt that repeated joint injury promotes osteoarthritis, the "wear and tear" arthritis. Vaccinations cause joint pain in some children[19] and adults[20]. Even medications contribute to some arthritis types. The classic NSAID treatment for osteoarthritis promotes joint destruction over a long period of time[6]. Estrogen replacement therapy, used by many women to offset menopausal symptoms, actually increases risk of developing systemic lupus erythematous[21]. There are even illnesses, like Lyme disease, that can mimic arthritis[22].

Sometimes, arthritis treatment involves complex detective work on the part of you and your doctor. While improving the quality of foods you eat will undoubtedly help your arthritis—85 percent or better are said to benefit from diet changes—don't ignore other causes.

All too often, long term use of such medical treatments as steroid drugs or gold injections can cause irreparable bodily harm. However, in the great majority of cases, you can expect at least some relief and perhaps a complete remission of arthritis symptoms for as long as you continue to avoid arthritis-aggravating foods and stay faithfully, instead, with a health-restoring diet.

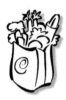

Ralph A. Stays Gout-Free with Restorative Foods

Ten years of discussing business deals over rich lunches and dinners left 45-year-old Ralph A. with sharp, stabbing gout pains in his big toes, insteps, and ankles. Seldom was more than a single joint attacked at one time, and the swelling and tenderness were excruciating.

On the advice of a nutritionist, Ralph cut out all seafood, meat, refined foods, caffeine and alcohol and replaced them with health-restoring natural foods. Gradually, the hot, shiny purple flesh around his afflicted joints turned to a healthy pink and Ralph's pains disappeared.

One day, a friend persuaded Ralph to try some anchovies and sardines on toast served with wine—all notorious gout-causing foods. Ralph thought that a single dietary indiscretion would hardly make a difference.

How wrong he was! By the following evening his left big toe began to throb and Ralph was right back where he began. Since then, Ralph has stayed strictly away from all gout-promoting foods. That was four years ago, and he has been free of all flare-ups and gout symptoms since.

Restorative Foods Work for Life

Ralph's experience is vitally important. To remain free of the symptoms of gout or arthritis—as well, probably, as those of other degenerative diseases—*you absolutely must stay with restorative foods for the rest of your life.* If you stray back to your old health-destroying foods, even for a snack, you may experience a sudden flare-up. Or you may wake up next morning to find that all the old stiffness has returned to your joints.

This may not mean having to give up *all* of your favorite foods forever, of course. But it does mean you should add more variety to your diet. If any favorite food is identified as provoking your arthritis, you may still be able to eat it provided you eat it less often and eat a variety of other health-restoring foods in between. Yet some foods are so harmful, they should never be eaten again.

As the Arthritis Foundation correctly states, arthritic disease cannot be cured. But you can decrease symptoms and even keep it in complete and permanent remission for the rest of your life.

Essentially, what this book does is to reveal the secrets by which one-in-ten people have helped their rheumatoid arthritis. The same secrets promise remission from all forms of arthritic disease.

Cure or remission? What difference what we call it provided you can lead a normal, active, pain free life without a trace of the symptoms of arthritis.

Within the limitations just described, you can take control of your health and arthritis, and still enjoy eating.

Regeneration of Joints by Restorative Foods

As the natural approach to healing has demonstrated, the more powerful your faith and expectation that you will recover, the better your chance for a speedy recovery. For as the natural rationale proves, nutrition is a critical factor in sound physical, mental, and emotional health.

The Six Recovery Steps are your beginning to better health and more manageable arthritis. Many people have reported a complete disappearance of arthritis symptoms within a week or so. For others it may take several weeks. In other cases, relief may be partial or more gradual.

Much depends on which type of arthritis you have. Rheumatoid and similar forms of arthritis often respond well to a change in diet, while recovery from gout may take a bit longer, and recovery from osteoarthritis may be very gradual.

How about structurally deformed bones and joints? No nutritional therapist can promise miracles. Through nutritional therapy you can end pain and regain joint mobility. But badly deformed joints may never regenerate completely. Nonetheless, you will have put a stop to further damage.

Yet among those one-in-ten people who permanently recover from that most crippling of arthritic diseases, rheumatoid arthritis, amazing examples of regeneration have occurred.

Never forget that the body is self-healing. It wants to get well. As your nutrition improves, your circulation will improve also. The rich body-building nutrients from the restorative foods which should now comprise your entire diet are carried into the bloodstream to nourish damaged muscle, bone, and tissue.

People who continue to make their health a primary concern often do experience a noticeable renewal or regeneration in arthritis-damaged joints. Gradually, as cells divide and renew themselves, structural joint damage may slowly improve.

George R. Puts His Own Body's Restorative Powers to Work

A case in point concerns George R. of Denver, Colorado. For nearly a decade, George suffered crippling rheumatoid arthritis in his ankles and toes. Eventually, his toes became so deformed that the joints spread haphazardly in all directions.

On the advice of a local masseur, George switched to a diet of fresh, natural restorative foods. Within three months, all pain and swelling had gone and George could walk almost as well as before.

But his toes continued to display bulging joints and they still spread randomly in all directions. After three years of eating nothing but health-building foods, coupled with regular daily walks and special toe and ankle activities, George's toes had noticeably improved.

Distortion and deformity still remain. But for all practical purposes, at age 52, George is fully recovered. In the more than three years during which he has stayed religiously with natural foods, he has not experienced a single flare-up.

We don't claim miracles. But, if you understand the principles of the natural approach to healing; if you continue to give your body the optimal chance to heal itself, then some degree of renewal and regeneration of deformed joints is a distinct possibility.

The Food You Eat Controls Your Health More Than Your Doctor Can with Drugs

Depending on your doctor's knowledge and attitude, you may still be told that using diet to improve arthritis is medically unsound.

If you are among the relatively few arthritis sufferers who, for one reason or another, nutritional therapy cannot help, the worst you have done is to spend the price of this book.

In return, you will have upgraded your nutrition to where it cannot fail to improve your overall health. According to the best consensus of medical and U.S. Government opinion, you will have significantly reduced your risk of contracting heart disease, hypertension, diabetes, and most of the other degenerative diseases that plague Americans.

Of course, no one can absolutely guarantee that any particular therapy will work for everyone. Your doctor certainly gives no guarantee that his medication will ease your pain and leave no side effects. What we do say is that the therapies in this book worked well for the people in the case histories and for scores of others whose stories could not be printed due to lack of space.

A Beginning Guide to Feeling Well

As you alter your eating habits to overcome arthritis, let your symptoms and instincts steer you. For the information and suggestions expressed in this book are *general guidelines, not individualized treatment*. This book is offering a basic plan to help arthritis, but you must fine tune your eating to suit your personal physical needs.

As rheumatology researchers make strides linking arthritis to diet, those in the natural medical field are refining their nutritional knowledge. We now understand that where and how you live, ethnic and cultural background, genetic make-up, and individual physiology all shape dietary need.

Restorative Foods May Save You Money

Most of the restorative foods we recommend are not exotic or expensive but are available in the produce department of your local supermarket. Most people find these foods often cost less than the affluent high fat foods they may be eating now.

A few restorative foods are available only in health food stores though that is changing. As we all become aware of how food affects health, consumer demand has forced regular grocery stores to carry some healthier foods. But no food costs as much as a visit to a doctor's office or the cost of filling the average prescription. Tens of thousands of people have spent their life's savings on conventional medical treatment for arthritis and have simply become worse. Some have died.

So if all you are getting from conventional treatment is bills, disappointments, and side effects, you owe it to yourself to read on and learn more about the amazing healing powers of restorative foods.

Chapter ***3***

How to Gain Power

Over Arthritic

Diseases

Knowing all about arthritis and its causes gives you a feeling of confidence and power over the disease. You realize you are no longer helpless and uninformed. Your health is in your own hands and your life is under your control.

Learning Everything About Arthritis Helps Carl S. Make a Complete Recovery

Carl S., an insurance salesman, had suffered from severe headaches for over five years. During the summer of his thirty-fifth year, the headaches became so bad he had to spend six weeks in bed in a darkened room.

X-rays revealed the culprit as rheumatoid arthritis. Heavy calcium deposits in Carl's spine and shoulder joints were pinching a nerve and causing the headache. Carl's doctor told him the disease was progressively degenerating, and within a few years he would be totally incapacitated.

Carl's wife, a dental assistant, was familiar with medical and nutritional literature. The couple spent the entire month of August studying everything available on rheumatoid arthritis. They soon concluded that pessimistic medical advice simply slams the door on self-help and the will to live and recover.

"As soon as I learned that arthritis was not something that attacks us from outside, I felt a tremendous feeling of power over the disease," Carl said. "I realized that neither drugs nor anything outside me was going to help. I could choose to recover by simply changing my diet."

On September first Carl did change his diet. Throughout their ten years of marriage, he and his wife had lived on canned and convenience foods with almost no fresh, natural produce. They replaced the cans and packages with whole, fresh natural foods.

Within three weeks, Carl's headaches and back pain had disappeared. Gradually, his joints were freed and movement restored. But by mid-November Carl was back at work. And he was soon practicing the flexibility exercises of yoga and tai chi to restore suppleness.

Still on his diet of natural foods at age 40, Carl has never felt better and he has experienced no arthritis flare-ups at all.

Natural Medicine—The Therapy of Tomorrow

Much of the knowledge we now have about arthritic disease has stemmed from research into immuno-therapy for cancer. A multiplicity of studies have found that nutrition affects immunity and thereby affects the potential for developing cancer and other degenerative diseases like arthritis.

Arthritis or more accurately, rheumatic disease, is the umbrella name for over 100 different diseases, syndromes, and conditions. The majority are nonarticular ailments which involve only soft tissue and not a joint. These include tendonitis and bursitis, often mild diseases in which medical care is seldom sought.

Most really painful varieties of arthritis are classified as articular types—meaning they affect a joint. Osteoarthritis is a "wear and tear" disease while gout is caused by excessive uric acid deposits, often resulting from rich food and drink. Fibromyalgia, the second most common type of arthritis, consists of generalized pain and tender muscle points. (See Chapter 17 for more details.) If we exclude these three for a moment, many of the remaining rheumatic diseases have a striking fact in common.

Almost every branch of medical science now recognizes them to be autoimmune diseases, caused by malfunctioning of the body's own immune system.

Autoimmunity is a situation in which the white cells of our immune system turn on the body's own tissue and attack it. In the light of this important discovery, let's briefly review the most common forms of arthritis and how each is caused.

Rheumatoid Arthritis: Currently 2,100,000 U.S. Cases

The most crippling form of arthritis, rheumatoid arthritis is most common in women aged 20–50; it also strikes older men. Target areas are the same joints of the hands and wrists and the knees; also the shoulders, ankles, elbows, neck, and spine. Joints in the hands and feet may become distorted and deformed, while the knees may become swollen with fluid. Afflicted joints are swollen, hot, tender, and extremely painful.

Rheumatoid arthritis is a systemtic disease affecting the entire body and is often accompanied by weight loss, poor appetite, fever, fatigue, and anemia. Rheumatoid nodules (lumps) may appear under the skin. Usually more than one joint is affected, and often pairs of joints become stiff and inflamed. The disease progresses in a series of flare-ups and remissions which may extend for months or even years.

In severe cases, joints may become fused and rigid. Approximately one fourth of all rheumatoid arthritis victims display "Sjögren's Syndrome" which results in difficulty in swallowing, dryness of nose, blanching of fingers, dry skin and eyes, vaginal dryness, and kidney afflictions.

Approximately one person in ten with rheumatoid arthritis experiences a complete and permanent remission and the disease never returns. A juvenile form called Still's Disease afflicts children, but approximately 80 percent of the victims recover completely.

Scientists consider both rheumatoid arthritis and Sjögren's Syndrome to be autoimmune conditions.

Ankylosing Spondylitis: Currently 318,000 U.S. Cases

This chronic inflammatory disease (also called Marie-Strümpell Disease) traditionally hits men aged 20–30. But since 1970, women of the same age are becoming increasingly susceptible. It is rare after 40.

Ankylosing spondylitis characteristically begins at the sacroiliac joints and creeps slowly up the spine. Hips, neck, and shoulders may become involved, and inflammation may occur in the eyes (uveitis), heart, and intestines in which case medical treatment should be sought.

But, usually only the spine is involved. Typically, the spine gradually curves forward until it eventually becomes calcified and fixed in a rigid curve. Or it may become ramrod-straight. However, symptoms are often much milder. After several years, pain and inflammation gradually subside and the victim is typically left with a permanent curvature of the spine.

Ankylosing spondylitis should be properly diagnosed and any lifesaving emergency treatment carried out. Some natural therapists believe the disease cannot be reversed after a person has had it for five years.

Like many forms of arthritis, ankylosing spondylitis is often triggered by an injury to the target area. Indicative of the role of the immune system in causing ankylosing spondylitis is that over 90 percent of people with the disease have the antigen HLA-B27 in their bloodstream. The B27 antigen also frequently exists in victims of other forms of arthritis, but it is found in only 5–8 percent of the general population.

Anyone with this genetic tendency towards autoimmunity has a significantly greater risk of contracting ankylosing spondylitis.

Systemic Lupus Erythematous (SLE)

SLE is a chronic inflammatory disease that strikes connective tissues throughout the body. Victims are characteristically women aged

15–40—female hormones are thought to influence this ailment. African-American and Hispanic women are affected more than whites. Men are also occasional victims. Symptoms appear slowly and range from weight loss and fatigue to hair loss (it grows back later), blanching of fingers, mouth ulcers, enlarged spleen and lymph nodes, joint pain and inflammation, and kidney involvement (which can be fatal).

A red butterfly-shaped skin rash on the face appears in half of patients. Many people have a mild form of SLE for which standard treatment involves rest as needed, no or few drugs, and emotional support. Spontaneous remissions and relapses are common. For others SLE is a serious disease that requires any vitally necessary medical treatment. But as this was written, no cure exists.

SLE is intimately connected with the body's endocrine system and immune system. Approximately 10–12 percent of all SLE cases are actually *pseudolupus* and are caused by drugs prescribed by doctors treating other diseases. Pseudolupus can be produced in scientific experiments by overloading the immune system with toxic drugs. When the drugs are withdrawn, the disease disappears. Flare-ups frequently occur when the immune system is overloaded by infections or by drugs such as sulfasalazine.

Here is a medically proven example of arthritis symptoms that are caused by ingested toxins and arthritis that disappears as soon as the toxins are removed from the body.

It is well established that SLE is an autoimmune disease.

Scleroderma

Scleroderma, also called progressive systemic sclerosis (PSS), is a slow moving systemic disease that strikes at connective tissue throughout the body. It appears in women two to three times as often as in men and usually begins between ages 35–55.

Symptoms begin with a dry, wax-like hardening and thickening of the skin. The skin tightens across the face and joints. PSS may spread to the blood vessels and muscles and to a variety of internal organs such as the heart, lungs, kidneys, and the digestive tract. Fingers, wrists, ankles, and knees may also be afflicted. The skin may become tight, swollen and dry, and swallowing may become difficult.

The first symptoms of this mystifying collagen disease is frequently Raynaud's phenomenon in which the hands turn purple and become dotted with white spots when exposed to cold. Currently, scleroderma is medically incurable but is fatal only if it afflicts a vital organ.

Scientists record that environmental exposure to toxins may prompt scleroderma[23].

PSS is diagnosed by examining the blood for characteristic antibodies and is considered a disorder of autoimmunity.

Other Diseases and Disorders

Other connective tissue disorders include polyarteritis nodosa, or inflammation of the blood vessels throughout the body and dermatomyositis, a systemic disease of the skin, muscles, and connective tissue which typically strikes women over 40. All are generally believed to be due to autoimmunity.

Rheumatic fever, once a dreaded childhood disease, can now be controlled by antibiotics. However, its decline began before the introduction of medicine, due to better health conditions—including nutrition. Rheumatic fever is believed to be triggered by an immunological reaction to strep infection—*meaning that it, too, may have an autoimmune connection.*

Thus far, all these common forms of arthritis have been scientifically determined to be autoimmune in nature, a dysfunction of our own white blood cells. And crippled digestion and food allergies may be at the bottom of it all.

Osteoarthritis: (Degenerative Joint Disease) U.S. Cases[24] Currently 20 Million

This most widespread form of arthritis usually appears after age 40–50 and afflicts two to three times as many women as men. Although your doctor will probably say that osteoarthritis is a "wear and tear" disease, it's not as simple as that. In the long ago days of intense physical labor and unrefined foods, osteoarthritis existed because bodies got used a lot and wore down. Unless you're involved in regular backbreaking physical work this probably won't happen to you. There's no doubt that elderly joints are also susceptible to erosion. But worn out joints aren't just the result of aging.

Nutrition is behind many osteoarthritis cases. This is borne out by the fact that the typical osteoarthritis victim is a heavy, overweight woman or man. People usually become obese after years of eating cooked, processed foods high in fat, sugar, white flour, and excessive animal protein. These same foods deprive the body of such essential nutrients as vitamins C and D and the B-complex and calcium, all of which are essential in the production of strong, healthy bone, and collagen. (Collagen is part of the connective tissue and cartilage in joints.)

Without these and other vital nutrients, the bone, cartilage and other tissue in joints become weak and easily damaged. Not only that, but without proper nutrition the body can't repair crumbling joints. Many people with osteoarthritis also suffer from a bone-weakening condition called osteoporosis in which the bones become thin, weak, porous, and brittle due to lack of calcium. Devastating free radical molecules, produced both by our own bodies to fight disease and in response to drugs and alcohol, encourage joint degeneration. When you eat foods rich in free radical squelching nutrients called antioxidants, this is less of a problem[25].

Now when such weight-bearing joints as those in the spine, hips, and knees are burdened with carrying the extra weight of an obese person, these nutritionally weakened joints break down and we have what is commonly called osteoarthritis. Years of inferior nutrition so depletes the bone, tissue, and cartilage in weight bearing and other joints that they become easily damaged by wear and tear. And as this same inferior nutrition creates obesity in the victim, a vicious circle ensues in which increasing body weight places increasing wear and tear on nutritionally weakened joints.

This is why the weight-bearing joints in the spine, knees, and hips are most commonly afflicted. But shoulders, elbows, wrists, and the ends of fingers may also be afflicted. Since osteoarthritis is not a systemic disease, damage is usually restricted to afflicted joints. Pain is usually moderate, stiffness more common than inflammation, and the disease is seldom crippling.

But if the hips are afflicted, it *can* lead to total and permanent disability, usually remediable only by installation of an artificial hip joint. Osteoarthritis is also called hyperthropic or degenerative arthritis. A mild variety, which usually strikes women under 40, causes bony protuberances on the end joints of fingers (Heberden's nodes).

Osteoarthritis is often triggered by a severe strain or injury or by overuse. This leads to a condition of stress in the joint cartilage—a rubbery cushion of protective tissue—causing it to lose its elasticity. As degeneration progresses, the cartilage may wear away, baring the bone joint surfaces and leaving them exposed to grind and grate against each other.

The body attempts to heal this distressed area with new cartilage around the joint edges. But all too often these calcify into hard, knobby spurs that interfere with joint mobility. Small pieces of bone may break off and grind in the joints. In severe cases, the entire inner bone construction of the joint can disintegrate and become deformed and distorted. Joints often have a knobby, misshapen appearance and muscles are weak.

Osteoarthritis is not considered to be caused by autoimmunity. Nonetheless, joint damage from pre-existing rheumatoid arthritis can lead to osteoarthritis. Healthy joints also depend on a healthy gastrointestinal tract. Sometimes treating food allergies, which may develop when the gut is ailing, improves osteoarthritis and joint pain.

But recovery usually requires as-needed rest combined with nutrient-rich restorative foods, a strongly positive attitude, and eliminating those factors that destroy cartilage and bone like NSAID drugs and inactivity. Together, this combination will rebuild weakened bone and cartilage, and gradually lead to optimal recovery and regeneration.

Gout: *Currently One Million U.S. Cases*

Gout is a metabolic (degenerative) disease caused by an elevated uric acid level in the blood. The typical victim is an overweight, sedentary male—men are twenty times as liable to develop gout as women. Although gout runs in families and may be due to a genetic tendency that leads to improper metabolism of purines in food, to overindulge in rich food and drink definitely invites the problem.

Each time someone indulges in life-wrecking foods, the victim's uric acid is overproduced and it precipitates on cartilage in the joints. Needle-like crystals of uric acid form and settle in joints, kidneys, and other tissue—though the big toe is the primary target area.

Although Hippocrates described gout 2,500 years ago, the actual process by which gout creates pain and inflammation was only discovered in 1981 as a result of a study by Dr. Gerald P. Rodnan of the University of Pittsburgh. Reportedly, Dr. Rodnan's study showed that uric acid crystals flake off joints and float in the synovial fluid that lubricates the joint. They are then recognized as foreign substances by the immune system and attacked by white cells.

But the crystal's sharp points pierce and kill these large white cells called phagocytes. As phagocytes die by the thousands, they release the same super powerful enzymes from their lysosome sacs as in the case of rheumatoid arthritis (the process of which is described later in this chapter). From there on, the process is almost identical with that of rheumatoid arthritis.

The body produces prostaglandins and other inflammatory substances to defend the joint against the flood of poisons released by the impaled phagocytes. As the prostaglandins begin the healing process, the afflicted joint becomes hot, swollen, and exquisitely tender. Gout is the most painful form of arthritis. Other joints, usually in the lower extremities, may also be affected. Kidneys unable to effectively excrete uric acid may form extremely painful kidney stones.

As increasing amounts of uric acid crystals are deposited around the joints, pain becomes sharp and stabbing, while irritation, scarring, and inflammation become severe.

Nature Forgives No Transgressions

If the victim continues to indulge, uric acid stones may appear in the urinary tract and eventually the kidneys can be damaged and destroyed.

The symptoms of gout are swelling, redness, and tenderness in the target joint often accompanied by a low fever. Over the joint, the flesh is often hot, shiny, and reddish-purple. Mild attacks may last only a few days, but more severe attacks can go on for weeks.

Today, gout can be stopped and controlled by drugs, though some drugs are very toxic and at the very least unpleasant. Steroids are often prescribed, but their use may lead to impotence. Too, gout often appears as a side effect of antihypertensive medication. Gout is also often associated with heart disease or hypertension and can be triggered by stress. Perhaps most surprising, aspirin, a recommended gout treatment[26], decreases uric acid excretion. This raises uric acid blood levels and can cause secondary gout[24].

Nonetheless, an avoidable cause of gout is a diet rich in purines which occur in such foods as alcohol, some fish, meat extracts, and organ meats.

A blood uric acid test taken by a physician can be used to diagnose gout, but levels can be high when symptoms are absent. Or you can be squirming in pain and have perfectly normal uric acid levels. Physical exam, medical history, and an aspiration of the afflicted joints by your doctor are more certain ways to confirm gout.

Because kidney damage can occur, it's important to control gout. Conventional medicine offers the drug colchicine, pain killers, bed rest, and dietary advice. If you prefer a natural approach, enlist the services of a qualified practitioner who's fluent in nutrition, herbs, and other safe, effective therapies.

As uric acid crystals are precipitated in the synovial fluid of the target joint, they create a highly stressful condition. Over-indulgence in rich, fatty foods creates the obesity that leads to the body's inability to deal with prolonged exposure to uric acid. Then certain foods aggravate the inflammatory reaction that often worsens the disease and makes it unbearable.

Sex, Age, and Arthritis

What science is saying about all of these forms of arthritis is that many are the result of or are intensified by autoimmunity. And autoimmunity, in turn, may relate to an ailing intestine and an allergy to one or more foods.

While food is an underlying exacerbator of most types of arthritis, the disease itself is often triggered by emotional stress, a physical injury, an illness, or an infection. Many researchers believe this is why certain arthritic diseases usually strike one sex more than another and are most common in certain age brackets.

Rheumatoid arthritis and lupus, for example, tend to affect women during the high stress childbearing years when a woman's immunity is lower before or after pregnancy or during certain stages of her menstrual cycle. On the other hand, most women with rheumatoid arthritis experience a remission during pregnancy because of depressed body defenses, including immunity against her own joints. Likewise, ankylosing spondylitis most frequently occurs in young men following an athletic injury. Too, emotional stress often sends a person heading for the refrigerator to find solace in fatty or sugary foods. Studies also show that rheumatoid arthritis often appears after an infection or cold, when immune system overload may activate autoimmunity in a susceptible person.

Knowledge Gives Larry A. Confidence in His Own Self-Healing Powers

Sometimes, even with the aid of modern lab tests, doctors have trouble diagnosing exactly which type of arthritis a patient may have.

Larry A.'s doctor could not decide whether the pains in his feet were caused by gout or arthritis. He prescribed 10 aspirins a day and told Larry to come back in six months when the disease would be sufficiently advanced to show up in blood tests.

For the next six weeks, Larry suffered continual agony. Finally, a friend recommended that he see a naturopathic physician. The naturopathic doctor explained that exact diagnosis wasn't essential since all forms of arthritis could be helped by nutritional therapy. He ordered Larry to exclude all types of processed foods and to eat only whole, fresh natural foods.

The realization that someone knew enough to recommend a therapy gave Larry a tremendous feeling of confidence in his own powers of recovery. He followed the naturopathic doctor's advice to the letter. In place of his former fast food meals and sugar-filled snacks, Larry began eating delicious salads of fresh fruits and vegetables.

Four weeks later, Larry was able to walk without pain. In the four years since, Larry has never strayed from his diet which he has now come to love.

Larry never did find out whether he had gout or rheumatoid arthritis. But one thing is certain: Since he gained enough power over his disease to totally overcome it, Larry has not had a single symptom.

See Your Doctor First

Because of possible complications caused by drugs or by other diseases, you should have a physical examination and obtain a diagnosis for any type of recurring arthritis type symptom or pain. In cases of connective tissue disease and other less common forms of arthritis, immediate medical treatment may be required to prevent damage to eyes and other organs. Many skilled alternative practitioners are available and can tell you if natural therapies are appropriate for your particular condition. (See Appendix C: Looking for a natural health practitioner.)

The nutritional therapy described in this book is not a substitute for essential medical treatment. If you have any life-threatening form of arthritis, you should have your doctor's approval before undertaking any suggestions in this book.

The natural therapies described in this book are suggested only when all emergency medical treatment is over and the patient has been pronounced permanently out of danger.

Stressor Foods Pave the Way for Arthritic Disease

Arthritis begins with the standard American diet—SAD for short because of the sorry state of most people's meals. Today, the average American derives 40 percent of his calories from fat and 22 percent from refined carbohydrates (white sugar, white flour, white rice). In fact, a recent survey of New York City supermarkets indicated that five of the 10 top "edible items" bought were soda pop products. Other popular purchases included beer, white sugar, and coffee[27].

Almost two-thirds of the calories most of us eat consists of just two foods—fat and refined carbohydrates. A similar flabby, health-threatening diet is eaten in other western industrial nations. So it should come as no surprise to learn that the U.S. has the world's highest rate of arthritic disease, with other western nations close behind.

By contrast, incidence of arthritis—and most other degenerative diseases—is many times lower in those third world countries where traditional foods like whole grains and legumes are staples.

Most Americans Are Overfed but Undernourished

As we continue to eat refined carbohydrates and fats along with frozen, canned, processed, and overcooked foods, a condition of marginal nutrition gradually builds up. Our bodies become increasingly deficient in such essential nutrients as vitamins A, C, D, E, and B-complex, and in such vital minerals as calcium, magnesium, manganese, potassium, and zinc.

Nutrients in foods we do eat often fail to be properly digested and absorbed due to less enzymes consumed, required for digestion. Raw foods contain some enzymes used for digestion. But since many enzymes in foods are destroyed by cooking, the extensive array of enzymes needed to digest cooked foods must be drawn from the digestive system alone.

Counterfeit Foods Upset the Body's Systems

The enzyme and nutrient deprivation of the typical American diet leaves every cell, tissue, and organ in the body nutritionally depleted. Particularly is this true of the pancreas which produces insulin so the body can use carbohydrates, and the liver which stores and metabolizes carbohydrates. To replace the enzymes lost in cooking, the pancreas must work overtime to manufacture digestive pancreatic enzymes. The pancreas must also produce extra insulin to offset the excessive fat in the American diet. (Fat inhibits the work of insulin in helping the body's cells to take up and utilize blood sugar. As a result, fat has been implicated along with refined carbohydrates as a major cause of maturity-onset diabetes.)

When people live on a nutritionally deficient diet, high in fats and sugar and low in natural enzymes and fiber, over a period of years their liver and pancreas suffer and become fatigued.

The extent of stress caused by living mainly on cooked foods was demonstrated in a study by Professor Schroeder of the Mayo Foundation when he made a study of Malays and Filipinos who lived exclusively on a diet of cooked foods. Their pancreases weighed 25–50 percent more than those of people who receive a natural supply of enzymes from vegetables, salads, and raw fruits.

Cooking and processing foods also alters their make-up and molecular structure, for instance creating more free radical molecules[28].

However, as Dr. Lisa Meserole, a naturopathic physician also trained in dietetics points out, cooking foods is not all bad. As with all aspects of nutrition, some people do well eating, say, half of their foods cooked. Others thrive on a mostly raw foods diet. Bowel diseases like Crohn's demand well cooked foods during inflammatory flare-ups; after this, raw foods can be slowly reintroduced into meals.

What is certain is cooking all or most of your food will deprive your liver and pancreas, two of the body's most vital organs. Any imbalance in nutrition leads to stress and imbalance in each of the body's other systems.

It can trigger a failure in carbohydrate metabolism sparking diabetes in prone individuals. It can suppress the immune system, leaving the body defenseless against cancer and infections. And it can harm our life line, the gastrointestinal tract, which may lead to food allergies. Poor digestion and food allergies may in turn feed autoimmune tendencies—a condition in which the immune system, which is supposed to protect us, turns around and attacks your own joints to produce arthritis.

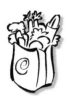 ## Marginal Nutrition Leads to Joint Distress

The glaring nutritional deficiencies of the typical American diet also leave the cells in our joints weak—unable to function properly or recover from everyday challenges. Wherever further stress is placed on a joint by injury, overuse or infection, it may be singled out for destruction by our equally overstressed immune system or merely lapse into disrepair.

Proof of the nutritional shortage in the typical American diet is the fact that a majority of arthritis sufferers have a deficiency of vitamins A, C, D, E, and the entire B-complex. In many arthritis patients, levels of vitamin C and B-complex are 50–75 percent below normal. Again, a serious calcium deficiency is almost standard, along with shortages of magnesium, manganese, potassium and zinc. Many people with arthritis also have a deficiency of food derived digestive enzymes as well as superoxide dismutase, an enzyme with free radical controlling properties. A severe imbalance in calcium-phosphorus-magnesium ratios is also common.

A well balanced level of each of these nutrients is necessary to supply the cells that maintain health in our joints.

Yet the foods we eat every day—the french fries, hamburger, apple pie, ice cream and coffee—are so lacking in essential nutrients and enzymes that they create stress and imbalance in every system in the body.

That is why we call these stressor foods. If you listed the foods most dangerous to health, every one would be a stressor food. These health-robbing foods have also been identified as contributing to *all* degenerative diseases, including heart disease, hypertension, diabetes, osteoporosis, and some forms of cancer.

Stressor foods also impair digestion and are responsible for some of our most common food allergies.

The first step in arthritis recovery is to ruthlessly eliminate these destructive foods from your diet—for the rest of your life.

Helen W.'s Newfound Power Helps Her Conquer Arthritis

Helen W. first had rheumatoid arthritis at age 42. For the next seven years, she took large daily doses of aspirin along with routine shots of cortisone. Several times a year, her knees would swell up so badly that her doctor had to drain out huge amounts of fluid by needle aspiration. Helen had pain so badly all over her body that she could sleep only when tranquilized.

One day, Helen read a book by a woman who had recovered from arthritis by eating only natural foods. The book described everything that was then known about arthritis and listed foods that experience showed caused flare-ups most often in the majority of people.

Helen found that this knowledge gave her such a newfound power that she felt confident and ready to act right away.

She decided that starting the next morning, she would eat only a single basic food each day such as milk, eggs, wheat, corn, sugar, beef, and chocolate. According to the book, if she experienced a flare-up it would be caused by her previous day's food.

This simple technique helped Helen identify sensitivities to milk, eggs, and sugar. After she had replaced these arthritis causing foods with fresh, natural foods, her pains gradually began to disappear. The swelling in her knees slowly returned to normal and eventually she was able to walk once more.

Now, five years later, Helen leads an active, pain-free life and sleeps soundly every night without pills.

Getting to the Stomach of the Problem

As stressor foods lower the body's overall health, two things happen. First, because our joints bear more physical stress than most other body parts, one or more joints may become distressed—degenerating faster than they can repair themselves.

Secondly, the nutritional deficiencies of stressor foods upsets our food metabolism process which, in turn, upsets our entire body chemistry. Each of the body's systems is thrown out of balance, but none more so than the vitally important gastrointestinal tract.

The gastrointestinal tract is your life line; without it you can't receive, digest, or absorb food. A crippled GI tract impairs nutrient delivery and every bodily process suffers.

Normally, digestion begins in the mouth as teeth chop food up and ptyalin, a starch-splitting enzyme, breaks food down. Food is then swallowed and shuttled to the stomach via the esophagus. Gastric juice contains enzymes, to smash apart protein and fat, and hydrochloric acid, to enhance mineral absorption and aid digestion.

The small intestine, an 18-foot muscular tube composed of the duodenum, jejunum, and ileum, receives stomach's predigested food. With help from enzyme-rich liquid from the pancreas, all major nutrients—fat, protein, and carbohydrates—are divided even further and most nutrients are absorbed. Bile, made by the liver but stored in the gallbladder, helps out with fat digestion too.

The GI tract ends with the five-foot colon, also called the large intestine. Here water and salts travel through its walls into blood vessels conserving water and electrolytes, and compact feces. This entire food trip takes anywhere from 12 to 24 hours.

When poor food selections, bad digestion, intestinal infections, drugs, disease, or surgery confront your gut, the rest of your body—including joints—suffer.

 ## Healthy Gut—Healthy You

A healthy intact intestinal tract is so important to your well-being because it's the only barrier separating you from the rest of the world. A barrage of food, germs, and chemicals—referred to as foreign antigens—pass through your gut everyday. If this 25-foot digestive tube breaks down at any point, these foreign particles infiltrate the rest of your body causing problems like arthritis.

Think of the intestine as a brick wall. Stressor foods, preservatives and additives, pesticides, even how you eat can loosen intestinal bricks and weaken your gastric fortress.

Low stomach acid and inadequate digestive enzymes pry apart the bricks of digestion. When mucous membranes and intestinal immunity fall apart, unwanted antigens sneak past cracks in the gut fence and into the bloodstream. Gastrointestinal diseases, like Crohn's and ulcerative colitis, and surgery create ongoing inflammation which further weakens the intestine.

Scientists admit autoimmune diseases, like rheumatoid arthritis, often arise when the intestine is unable to handle and process its daily load of antigens. Robert Inman, MD, professor of Immunology at the University of Toronto in Ontario, Canada, says GI tract performance varies depending not only on foreign antigen type, but how much of it we ingest, for how long and how often. Intestinal flora also shapes GI health[29].

A metropolis of 400 different species of friendly bacteria and other germs normally reside in a healthy gut. These neighborly organisms not only keep each other and bad bugs in check, but in return for their accommodations, produce vitamins and other beneficial compounds like natural antibiotics for you. Some strains even help fight cancer[30].

Normally the GI tract is well prepared to battle incoming germs with its arsenal of immune-active cells and battalion of congenial bacteria. However, when pathogenic germs overwhelm intestinal troops, called dysbiosis, your intestinal barricade weakens. Included among the microbial foe are Candida, a type of yeast, and parasites.

The Food Allergy-Arthritis Connection

We can't say that food allergies cause arthritis in everyone. We can't even say that food allergies initiate all instances of arthritis. What is clear, according to recent research, is the link between food sensitivity and joint inflammation in some people.

In their comprehensive 1991 review entitled "Rheumatoid Arthritis, Food, and Allergy" (*Seminars in Arthritis and Rheumatism*), Drs.

van de Laar and van der Korst state an unhealthy bowel and various arthritis types often go hand-in-hand. As many as two-thirds of those with rheumatoid arthritis are plagued by a stomach complaint called chronic atrophic gastritis. Rheumatoid arthritis sufferers are frequently plagued with low stomach acid too[28].

To fully understand food allergies, we must endure a quick lesson in immunology.

The immune system is the body's resistance against disease. It is a network of billions of tiny roving white cells that patrol the bloodstream to seek out and destroy invading foreign cells, viruses, bacteria, and other particles.

The white cells can be compared to defending soldiers. White cells called lymphocytes are biologically programmed to attack and destroy not only foreign invaders but also cancer cells and any body tissue that is badly run down, weakened by stress such as physical injury, toxic build-up, or overuse.

Phagocytes are large white cells that mop up after a lymphocyte attack. Within their cell membranes are sacs of highly destructive enzymes called lysosomes. (These metabolic enzymes are different from digestive enzymes.) After a lymphocyte attack, phagocytes kill off any remaining enemy cells with their enzymes, then ingest the debris for destruction by their lysosomes.

A common dysfunction that occurs in the immune system is an allergy, an over-reaction to usually harmless substances like food and pollen. Allergy-prone individuals are born with genes programmed to kick the immune system into overdrive when a speck of food or dust invades. Particles of food are rejected in exactly the same way as are a transplanted heart or kidney. Their antigens are recognized as foreign.

 ## Non-Tolerated Food Particles Trigger Immune Reaction

This food rejectivity response varies with each individual. An allergy to, say, milk that may trigger arthritis in one person may trigger migraine in another.

No two people have identical body chemistry. Each of us may have our own unique reaction to a certain food. Also, most people with food sensitivities are allergic to several foods, not merely one. And at the bottom of multiple food intolerances is often a shaky GI tract.

The conventional medical establishment's disenchantment with nutrition as a cause of arthritis stems from the efforts of science to isolate one or more foods which are *invariably* responsible for arthritis. We now know that this is not possible because treating food allergies (and arthritis) requires more than removing the offending food. It requires rehabilitation of the digestive system and perhaps other lifestyle and therapeutic adjustments as well. Hence the Arthritis Foundation, as well as many doctors, continue to downplay the link between arthritis and diet or nutrition.

In reality, what happens is this: Every cell or virus is coated with a protein substance which carries a recognition code called an antigen. Lymphocytes patrolling the bloodstream recognize the antigen of every cell they meet as either "self" and friendly, or as "foreign" and hostile.

Immune Reaction Turns Cell Against Cell

Whenever a lymphocyte encounters a foreign invader, it immediately triggers a body-wide alarm. Killer lymphocytes migrate through the bloodstream to attack and neutralize the invader with toxic enzymes. Meanwhile, other lymphocytes manufacture antibodies, protein substances which recognize and attack the invader's antigen.

As we digest a meal, tiny particles of food—some only partly broken down—are absorbed through a sieve-like intestinal wall into the bloodstream. A healthy gastrointestinal tract is intact allowing mostly digested food molecules to pass through into circulation. Those with intestinal disease or allergies may have an overabundance of large food molecules crossing the intestinal threshold due to a condition called "leaky gut syndrome." Leaky gut describes the increased permeability or abnormal sieve-like nature of the intestine.

In 1995, British scientists communicated in the *Journal of the Royal Society of Medicine* (volume 88) what many natural health practitioners already suspected—24 of the 30 people they tested with food intolerances also had leaky guts[31]. In many cases, people with rheumatoid arthritis have more permeable guts than the arthritis-free. Sadly the very medicines used to treat osteoarthritis and rheumatoid arthritis, namely NSAIDs, also increase intestinal permeability[28].

A leaky gut is the epitome of intestinal barrier breakdown. For it's through these "holes" that noxious substances, normally barred from the body, sneak through. Problems magnify when poor digestion only partially breaks food down. Dysbiosis creates more havoc by interfering with digestion and creating its own brand of toxins.

Larger than normal food particles, that pass through a leaky gut, are recognized as foreign antigens and a food allergy is born. Chronic spilling of partially digested food, bacterial toxins and other vagabond molecules across the GI barrier can spark bizarre system-wide, immune behavior.

These are the foods and irritants that the body, in its nutritionally depleted state, is no longer able to tolerate. Usually, these are the very foods we eat most of. There's many explanations for this. Residues from pesticides, fertilizers, and other chemicals permeate our food and may initiate reactions to food. With the introduction of irradiation, pasteurization, and genetic engineering, some modern day foods are structurally different from those consumed years ago. As an example, Midwest scientists revealed that a strain of soybeans, genetically crossed with Brazil nuts, provoked immune responses in subjects known to be allergic to Brazil nuts *but not soybeans*[32].

The allergy that usually results is known as a delayed or hidden allergy. Unlike other allergies such as those caused by insect stings, dust, pollen, animal danders, and some foods (which produce instantly visible rashes, hives, or hayfever) delayed food allergies often produce symptoms body-wide.

Arthritis Happens When the Body Turns on Itself

The immune response to tiny particles of allergic food in the bloodstream is to recognize it as a foreign invader. A rejection response occurs exactly as if it were an infectious virus or bacterium.

Meanwhile, the entire lymphocyte population begins to multiply in great numbers. In a very short time, the white blood cell count soars just as during an infectious disease. Suddenly, the bloodstream is filled with armies of aggressive lymphocytes thirsting for battle.

In the genetically vulnerable the crazed immune system goes one step farther. Cross reactivity occurs where swarms of surplus lymphocytes zero-in not only on food specks, but also body proteins like those in joints. If that joint is also weak, all the better. This is called autoimmunity where lymphocytes and other immune factions recognize joint cells as foreign.

Here again, antibody manufacturing lymphocytes produce a barrage of antibodies that will recognize the joint cells' antigen and attack it.

Antibodies coupled with foreign antigens, called antigen-antibody complex, spew onto the already weakened joint cells. This toxic combination harasses the synovial membrane which secretes synovial fluid, the lubricant of body joints. It also eats away at the cartilage which cushions friction between moving bones. In SLE and scleroderma, the same antigen-antibody complex is considered responsible for damage to blood vessels, kidneys, and to the membranes of heart and lung.

The Autoimmune Reaction Is Now at Its Height

The body responds by increasing blood flow to the afflicted joint and produces healing prostaglandins. In its efforts to protect and heal itself, the joint becomes hot, red, inflamed, and painful. Large amounts of synovial fluid are secreted to protect the knee joints. This creates the common arthritic symptom of swelling in the knees. Swelling can become so severe that synovial fluid must be removed by needle aspiration.

As lymphocytes and antibodies conflict with antigens in the target joint, phagocytes move in to mop up. In what immunologists call a cytotoxic reaction, large numbers of phagocytes in the joint are poisoned by the antigen-antibody complex produced during the antigen-antibody clash.

.As thousands of phagocytes continually die in the target joint, their lysosomes collapse and super-powerful enzymes escape on to the already reeling tissue cells.

The body defends itself against the autoimmune attack by creating inflammation, swelling, stiffness, tenderness, heat, and pain in the afflicted joint.

This is how arthritis is born!

The Body Itself Creates Arthritis

Note carefully that the body itself creates arthritis. Arthritis symptoms were not created by autoimmune attack or by food allergies or by marginal nutrition or obesity or anything else.

The body itself creates arthritis symptoms in an attempt to defend itself from autoimmune attack and to promote healing.

Note, too, that gout symptoms are created by the body as it attempts to defend and heal itself against the destructive enzymes released by dying phagocytes.

Natural health philosophy says the body can create, the body can reverse. When the cause of disease is removed, the body becomes self-healing. When we heal the gut, cut out the stressor and allergy foods that lead to arthritis, and replace them with restorative foods that supply nutrients the body needs for self healing, then the body will heal itself.

The program in this book is based on this principle.

Remembering the Lessons of Health Cures Nancy M.'s Painful Knees

As a natural health physician, Nancy M., 43, knew the importance of proper eating. Yet with the pressures of a busy practice and family life, Nancy let her normally good diet slide.

Over a period of several months, Nancy noticed an aching in her knees and heels, something she'd never experienced before. She knew she didn't have arthritis, but suspected her poor meal choices, especially sweets, were to blame.

Unable to ignore the problem any more, Nancy began to cut out sweets and fats, and decrease her intake of wheat. She ate brown rice and steamed raw vegetables for ten days. Immediately after eliminating wheat, a suspected allergy food for her, and following a gentle body cleansing program, her joints and heels were fine. Stomach pains, something else that bothered her, also disappeared.

Arthritis—The Gut-Wrenching Disease

The arthritis causing process just described builds on itself in a vicious, self-perpetuating action for as long as we continue to eat gut wrenching and allergy-causing foods. Only by ceasing to eat the non-tolerated foods can we break the spiral of chronic degeneration.

Meanwhile, autoimmunity creates ever-increasing pain and dysfunction in the now arthritic joint. As the body struggles to maintain its self-healing efforts, bony spurs build up on the sides of bones and excess calcium is deposited around the target joint.

Besides causing degeneration in joints, autoimmunity affects the body in various secondary ways. In rheumatoid arthritis, it leads to fever, fatigue, weight-loss, depression, loss of appetite, and harm to various organs. And because we frequently crave allergenic foods, we eat them in such large amounts that they may cause headaches, indigestion, diarrhea, and other types of gastrointestinal upsets, of course related to an already ailing digestive tract.

While poor diet nudges the body toward painful arthritis, arthritis itself sabotages nutritional state. The physical limitations of arthritis make it difficult for many to shop for and prepare nutritious meals. Inflamed joints increase the body's metabolic rate so it burns up fuel and nutrients quicker than usual.

The GI-joint connection is a Catch-22. While indigestion exacerbates joint problems, gut troubles are also caused by arthritis. Either way, absorption and digestion of food diminishes, which further weakens ailing joints. Even arthritic medication depletes vitamins and minerals desperately needed by weakened joints[28].

As long as non-tolerated foods continue to be eaten, rheumatoid arthritis symptoms remain and intensify in the target joints. When a larger amount of non-tolerated foods than usual is consumed, a flare-up of the disease invariably follows.

When by accident or coincidence, one or more non-tolerated foods are eliminated, the disease often dies down. It may remain in remission until the non-tolerated foods are eaten again.

If they are never eaten again, the disease is likely to remain in remission indefinitely.

The second step in arthritis recovery is to repair the gastrointestinal tract; the third step requires identification of all allergy foods and to cut them completely out of your diet.

Chapter **4**

The Six Recovery Steps

for Overcoming

Arthritis

Gout, osteoarthritis, and rheumatoid arthritis are three totally different diseases. In each disease, different foods work in different ways to produce different symptoms.

Yet the basic recovery steps for all three diseases are quite similar.

The Six Recovery Steps

Recovery Step #1. *Cut out all stressor foods* (Chapters 10 and 11). Stressor foods are those health-robbing junk foods that undermine the body and set the stage for joint problems. Insufficient nutrients weaken joints thus impinging repair efforts. Bad diet creates a leaky gut that leads to food allergies and possibly autoimmune problems like rheumatoid arthritis. Poor food choices and inactivity causes excess weight which overburdens joints already suffering from marginal nutrition; the result, osteoarthritis. High uric acid levels, worsened by purine loaded foods, invites gout.

61

Recovery Step #2. *Repair the gastrointestinal tract with healthy eating* (Chapters 5 and 6). At the bottom of many food allergies, and possibly autoimmune disorders, is a sick digestive tract. Because a prime directive of natural medicine is to find and treat the root cause of health problems, healing the gut with sound eating practices is compulsory if you want to reverse arthritis.

Recovery Step #3. *Cut out all allergy foods* (Chapters 5, 7, 8, and 9). Rheumatoid and similar forms of arthritis (ankylosing spondylitis, lupus, scleroderma, etc.) occur when the immune system attacks the body's own joints and tissue. These attacks may be precipitated by partially digested particles of allergenic foods in the bloodstream. When we stop eating foods to which we are allergic, the immune system often ceases attacking our joint cells and tissue and the pain and swelling of arthritis gradually disappears.

Recovery Step #4. *Rebuild damaged joints and health with restorative Foods* (Chapters 12, 13, and 14). Restorative foods are nutrient-packed whole foods that the body needs to heal itself and restore health. When we heal our GI tract and stop eating all stressor and allergy foods, arthritis greatly improves. At this point, the body becomes self-healing. By eating restorative foods, we give the body the nutrients it needs to rebuild afflicted joints, the gut, and other tissues and to restore bowel regularity and good digestion.

Recovery Step #5. *Where overweight exists, gradually reduce it to normal* with weight-reducing restorative foods (Chapter 15). A return to normal weight is an essential step in complete recovery from gout or osteoarthritis. Natural foods high in fiber and low in fat create safe, comfortable, and gradual weight-loss without counting calories or feeling hungry.

Recovery Step #6. *Eliminate gastrointestinal stress by learning to eat properly.* All forms of arthritis are worsened by unwise eating practices. (We're talking about the way we eat, not food itself.) Chapter 16 describes how to upgrade eating techniques to eliminate most gastrointestinal complaints and the arthritic disease to which they are linked.

Maximizing Your Chances for Arthritis Recovery

An obese gentleman who had osteoarthritis along with chronic indigestion and constipation read an early draft of this book. He told one of the authors, "You'll be glad to know I've decided to cut out sugar and I'm adding bran to my diet."

That was all. No weight-reducing restorative foods. No improvements in the act of eating that could have eliminated his chronic indigestion. Nothing about cutting out fat-laden stressor foods.

A few months later, his constipation improved. But he was still seriously overweight and he still suffered from arthritis and chronic indigestion.

Token cooperation with just one or two steps isn't usually enough to overcome arthritis. If you're really earnest about recovering from arthritis, you must act fully and without reservation right now and go *all the way* into *all* the steps that affect you.

(If you're not overweight, or if your arthritis is *not* aggravated by food allergies, only five steps need to be taken. We'll get to these exceptions later.)

But to maximize your chances of recovery from arthritis as soon as possible, you should act right now on *all* the steps that personally affect you.

How to Get Started on the Recovery Steps

The way to get started is to read through the rest of this book as soon as you can. The following chapters flow right on into how to repair your gastrointestinal tract (Chapter 6); identify your allergy foods (Chapters 7, 8, and 9); how to cut out stressor foods

(Chapters 10 and 11); how to rebuild your health with restorative foods (Chapters 12, 13, and 14); and how to reduce weight with wholesome foods (Chapter 15). You should also read Chapter 16 which describes important eating techniques that can end gastrointestinal problems and hasten your recovery.

Check out other natural health techniques—besides diet—not covered in this book but nevertheless helpful for arthritis. For example, glucosamine sulphate is extremely useful in rebuilding worn out cartilage in osteoarthritis. If you have fibromyalgia, an up and coming rheumatic disease, take a look at Chapter 17.

While self care often works, enlisting a qualified natural health practitioner will improve your chances of recovery (See Appendix C).

Skim through these chapters first to get the overall picture and to learn how the recovery steps provide a thoroughly natural approach to helping arthritis. Then as you actually carry out each step, you should study the relevant chapters in detail.

Which Step Should You Act on First?

Ideally, you should get at least four steps under way as soon as possible. But as you'll probably put only one step into effect at a time, begin with Step 1. Begin by cutting out all stressor foods.

Step 2, repairing your GI tract, is vital because intestinal problems are what egg on many arthritis cases. Part of digestive recovery involves the 7-day Self Purification Technique (Chapter 5), also used to detect allergy foods. After that, you're ready to make dietary adjustments that heal and prevent further intestinal woes (outlined in Chapter 6).

In Step 3, you identify your own food allergies. The recommended way is to undergo a 7-day Self Purification Technique (Chapter 5) to prepare you for 10 days of subsequent food testing (Chapters 7 and 8). This system of identifying food allergies is called the elimination-challenge technique.

During the 10 days of food testing, you eat a single test food each day together with your already established healing diet. During these 10 days you should avoid any social eating where you might be pressured into contaminating the tests by taking another food or beverage.

What If You Can't Schedule All Steps Right Away?

The 7-day Self Purification Technique usually requires your taking off at least a day or two from work. So you may want to postpone the Self Purification Technique until a long weekend holiday or your next vacation.

Meanwhile, you can use alternative techniques for identifying food allergies described in Chapter 9. Some of these alternative methods aren't as sensitive nor do they give as positive a response as when using the Elimination-Challenge Technique. But you may very well be able to identify all or most foods which are aggravating arthritis without interrupting your busy lifestyle. Other suggested methods are laboratory tests requiring your doctor's help. These tests are less time consuming and taxing than the elimination-challenge method, and in some cases more accurate.

If you'd rather forgo expensive tests at this point, then at the first opportunity you can still undertake the Self-Purification Technique to ferret out any remaining food allergies you may have missed.

If it isn't convenient to put all steps into effect immediately, at least begin with Steps 1 and 4.

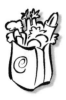

Astonishing Benefits from Excluding Stressor Foods

By taking Step 1 and cutting out all stressor foods, you immediately eliminate all the most harmful foods that you eat. Many stressor foods cause hardening of the arteries, constipation, gastrointestinal problems, obesity, and nutritional deprivation, and they disturb the balance of your body chemistry—all factors that may lead right into arthritis.

You may also be allergic to some stressor foods. When you act 100 percent on Step 1, you take a huge step towards better health and freeing yourself from arthritis. Then by taking Step 4, you replace all health-destroying stressor foods with health-building restorative foods.

Step 4 actually takes you halfway into Step 5—restoring your weight to normal with wholesome foods. And you can easily add Step 6—upgrading your eating habits—by reading Chapter 16.

How a Leaky Gut and Allergy Foods May Worsen Gout or Osteoarthritis

Now Steps 1, 4, 5, and 6 alone can help reverse gout or osteoarthritis provided it is uncomplicated by any rheumatoid component.

What is rheumatoid component?

Pure gout or osteoarthritis is not usually provoked by food allergies. Gout is aggravated by eating foods high in purines, the basic stuff of uric acid. Osteoarthritis is caused by the wear and tear of carrying excessive body weight.

So if you have either of these forms of arthritis, Step 3 isn't going to help all that much, although Step 2 may.

But, both gout and osteoarthritis may weaken cells in afflicted joints to the point where, if a food allergy exists, these joints may then become targets for autoimmune attack. This is called cross-reactivity where an allergy to a certain food crosses over to include joints too.

Autoimmunity may be triggered by food allergies, and in the run-down health condition that accompanies gout and osteoarthritis, some people *do* develop food allergies.

When this happens you may have rheumatoid-type pain, swelling, heat, and inflammation superimposed on the symptoms of osteoarthritis or of gout.

When rheumatoid symptoms are superimposed on osteoarthritis, you have what doctors often call "double arthritis." Both rheumatoid and osteoarthritis exist together.

Rheumatoid symptoms can superimpose on gout too.

If you have already been diagnosed as having osteoarthritis, you can easily tell if double arthritis develops because inflammation, heat, and swelling will appear in one or more joints. Normally, osteoarthritis is a fairly mild affliction which involves relatively moderate pain accompanied by stiffness rather than inflammation.

Recovery Steps for Gout

Since gout produces both excruciating pain and inflammation, the only way to tell if rheumatoid arthritis symptoms are also present is through lab tests. Rather than incur this expense, we suggest putting Steps 1, 4, 5, and 6 into effect first.

If after several weeks, no significant improvement appears, then consider taking Step 2 and 3. You should know, however, that the Self-Purification Technique will probably intensify gout symptoms rather than relieve them. This is because as the body detoxifies itself, stored-up uric acid crystals in the joints are broken down and released into the bloodstream where they immediately create gout pain and swelling.

Thus if you have gout, you or your doctor may prefer to test for food allergies by using laboratory methods described in Chapter 9.

Recovery Steps if You Are Overweight

Apart from setting off a gout flare-up (which should be only temporary), the Self Purification Technique is an excellent way to launch a weight-loss program, though fasting and food deprivation rarely lead to permanent weight loss. Anyone with an eating disorder should avoid fasting and cleansing programs without the careful supervision of a physician knowledgeable in these disciplines. Restoring your weight to normal is an essential step in total recovery from gout or osteoarthritis.

The use of wholesome foods to reduce weight to normal without crash dieting or counting calories is described in Chapter 15. Also, as you feel better you'll be more inclined to exercise, absolutely necessary to both maintain ideal weight and healthy joints.

The Recovery Step That May Bring Fast Pain Relief

Steps 2 and 3 are often the keys to recovering from rheumatoid and similar forms of arthritis aggravated by food allergies and poor intestinal health. Since overweight is seldom a problem in rheumatoid arthritis, Step 5 may be unnecessary. But Steps 1 and 4 are both vital to recovery and Step 6 is almost always required.

The heart of Steps 2 and 3 are the Self Purification Technique which frequently halts immune system attack on afflicted joints. Since autoimmune attack is the principal reason for pain and inflammation in rheumatoid and similar forms of arthritis, inflammation, swelling, and heat caused by autoimmune attack often subside while pain may even end altogether.

Observations have shown that 70 percent of arthritis pain (excluding gout) is temporarily benefited or even ended by the 7-day Self Purification Technique.

You should realize that it is *rheumatoid* arthritis pain and inflammation which Steps 2 and 3 help. In people with double arthritis or with gout, the rheumatoid pain and inflammation worsened by food allergies may subside. But the underlying gout or osteoarthritis may not benefit quite so soon.

Since in double arthritis the rheumatoid component is responsible for much of the pain, Steps 2 and 3 can obviously bring important relief. But it may not end pain and stiffness due to wear and tear. The osteo-component is helped by Step 4 which is a more gradual process.

Reading for Rapid Recovery

Because Steps 2 and 3 have proven to be the most direct way to benefit arthritis pain, many readers will doubtless wish to begin it as soon as possible. For this reason, it is described in Chapters 5, 6, 7, 8, and 9 which immediately follow.

Again, since you may be allergic to some stressor foods, a knowledge of food allergies is a prerequisite to reading more about Step One, stressor foods. Hence stressor foods are dealt with in Chapters 10 and 11.

We explain this apparent order of reversal to avoid misunderstandings. The fact that Step 1 is dealt with in later chapters in no way implies that you should postpone acting on Step 1.

Jenny K. Recovers from Arthritis When She Overcomes Her Own Inertia

How many arthritis sufferers will read the rest of this book then put it down and say, "I'm sure it's all very nice,"—and never do another thing about it!

If inertia and the comfort of familiar but bad eating habits is keeping you stuck in a rut, give yourself a big push and get started.

Jenny K. had rheumatoid arthritis for three years when she read a book published decades ago about a lady who had reversed arthritis with natural foods. Jenny found the book enthralling. But it asked her to make radical changes in her eating habits. Although Jenny realized she was eating poorly, she felt very comfortable with her familiar foods and beverages.

"Besides it probably wouldn't work for me, anyway," she consoled herself.

Then a friend called to tell Jenny about a wonderful course she had just taken in positive thinking. The friend explained to Jenny the various reasons why most people fail to live up to their good resolutions. When Jenny discovered how easy it actually was to psyche herself up to change her diet, she decided to go ahead immediately.

"Right away, I learned I must take responsibility for my own health," she said. "No thing or person can turn your health around and make you well. You have to do it yourself. I learned that it's never too late to start. And no matter how often you stray from your diet, don't be put off. Get right back into it again."

Jenny's friend told her not to expect a rose garden.

"She told me to be prepared for some discomfort," Jenny said. "She also advised me to set realistic goals. So instead of changing over to a 100 percent natural foods diet immediately, I increased the amount of natural foods in my diet by 20 percent each week. I found I could easily live with that."

The book Jenny was following simply advised cutting out all health wrecking foods and replacing them with fresh, natural foods. Gradually, week by week, as Jenny began to feel better, the improvement served as feedback to encourage her to continue. But despite the improvement, low residual pain and inflammation continued to linger on.

Jenny began reading more recent literature. She learned about food allergies and their link to arthritis.

"I self-tested several foods to which I suspected I was allergic," she said. "I found out I had allergies to wheat, corn and oats, all foods that the original book had said were O.K."

When Jenny removed these grains from her diet, improvement was dramatic. Within two weeks, the last of her pain and inflammation disappeared.

"That was two years ago and I haven't had a flare-up since," Jenny said. "I've stayed strictly with natural foods all the while.

Once I overcame my inertia and took charge of my life, I found it was a whole lot easier and more comfortable to change my diet and feel better than to go on doing nothing and continue to suffer pain."

Recovery Steps Can Supplement Conventional Medical Care

Another factor that may influence when and how you decide to take the steps to recovery is how well these Steps mesh with essential conventional medical care.

It is certainly not our intent to discourage you from taking any essential medication or undergoing any necessary medical treatment.

Using natural medical treatments don't cancel out conventional medical care. In fact, the two methods can be used simultaneously and complement one another. It's gratifying to see all medical practitioners—MDs, chiropractors, osteopaths, and naturopathic physicians—starting to work together to keep their patients well.

Some types of arthritis, especially those that afflict connective tissue, may endanger your eyes, heart or kidneys if not promptly treated. We certainly would not discourage anyone from taking any life-saving treatment or other essential emergency medical care, whether administered by an MD or competent naturopathic doctor.

However, when all danger is over and all emergencies are past, certainly consider the self-help therapies described in this book. If you are still under necessary medical treatment, you should certainly consult your doctor before making any changes in diet, undergoing the Self Purification Technique, testing foods, losing weight, or doing anything else that might have a deleterious effect on your health. Or you may need your doctor's help instigating some of these ideas.

How to Tell if Your Doctor Is Really Helping You

The problem is, however, that many conventional doctors are still so set against any alternative therapy that they will veto it automatically. If this is the case, your doctor may be doing you a real disservice.

If you suspect your doctor is prejudiced against alternative therapies, the solution is to change to another, more naturally oriented physician. Choose a modern doctor who looks ahead to safe health promoting therapies of the future instead of one who belongs to the backward looking cutting and drugging school.

Let your new doctor decide whether it is safe for you to practice an alternative therapy. Hopefully, your new physician will also take you off all but the most essential drugs.

Again, we urge that if you are under medical care, you consult your doctor before reducing any essential medication or making any dietary or other changes.

The solution is not to disobey your doctor. The answer is to change to a new physician who *will* cooperate and work with you, by allowing you to safely use the therapies described in this book. Even if that doctor knows nothing about natural medicine, but is open-minded enough to learn, then you're one step closer to recovery.

Shirley N. Triumphs Over Arthritis with Natural Therapies

Shirley N. had increasing pain and stiffness in her ankles, toes, wrists, and fingers. Swallowing became difficult and she suffered from almost continual gastrointestinal upset. After a series of lab tests, her doctor diagnosed progressive systemic sclerosis.

Scleroderma or PSS, as it's also called, is a slow but dangerous form of connective tissue disease. If not controlled, it causes progressive hardening of the skin, crippling of the fingers, and increasing damage to joints and internal body organs.

Shirley responded to medication, and progress of the disease seemed halted. But the drugs produced a variety of unpleasant side effects ranging from nausea to vomiting, diarrhea, and internal bleeding.

Meanwhile, Shirley had read everything available on alternative therapies for arthritic disease. She asked her doctor if she could change her diet and test herself for food allergies.

The answer was an emphatic "No!"

One day, Shirley noticed a sign that read, "Whole Person Health Center." Under it were the names of four MDs. Shirley immediately consulted one of the doctors who agreed to take her as his patient.

"Right off, the new doctor said that the drugs were only masking the symptoms of scleroderma," she said. "He said the only way to reverse it was to remove the cause. He was very enthusiastic about changing to a diet of natural foods and about testing for food allergies.

"My new doctor cut my medication to the barest minimum. Then he said I should go ahead with the Self Purification Technique for seven days.

"When he checked me on the seventh day, all my intestinal pains had cleared up and the pain and stiffness in my joints already felt better.

"My doctor okayed me for 10 days of food testing and he actually helped me do it. It was a new experience for him, too. Well, between us we decided I was allergic to sugar, milk, coffee, beef, pork, wheat, and potatoes. He said I had no business eating most of those foods to begin with. He told me to cut out a lot of other foods high in fat and refined flour and sugar.

"So I went on eating a diet of nothing but natural foods. Pretty soon I could swallow without discomfort. The swelling and inflammation in my fingers and toes were disappearing and the stiffness was leaving my other joints. About four months after I first changed to my new doctor, he pronounced a complete remission."

Her doctor warned Shirley that the remission would last only as long as she maintained sound nutrition and good health habits. As of this writing, insufficient time has elapsed to confirm the remission as permanent. But Shirley has obviously become a completely new person with a powerful desire to overcome all obstacles and to remain in optimum health for the rest of her life.

Yet as she herself said, "If I hadn't spotted that sign on the holistic health center, I'd have gone on being an invalid for life."

The Recovery Steps Are a Lifetime Program

As Shirley's doctor pointed out, she must stay with restorative foods for life. She must avoid eating stressor foods. However, in Chapter 16 you learn how you may be able to begin eating certain allergy foods later on by adding more variety to your diet.

Regardless of what type of arthritis you have or in what order you decide to begin the recovery steps, all stressor foods should be cut out as rapidly as possible and replaced with restorative foods.

For example, if you decide you must wait 10 days before commencing the Self-Purification Technique and food testing, you should try to put Steps 1 and 4 into effect just as soon as possible.

If you are reading this book slowly, say at the rate of a chapter every day or two, we recommend reading Chapters 10, 11, 12, and 13 first and acting on them to improve your diet as quickly as possible.

By doing so, you may even recover from arthritis before you finish reading this book. It *has* happened!

Chapter *5*

The Miracle Healing Technique That Banishes Most Arthritic Pain Within Seven Days

---

Imagine a simple do-it-yourself technique that you can practice at home without exercise and for minimal expense that in seven days will:

- End all or most of the pain of arthritis.

- Diminish heat and swelling in arthritic joints.

- Begin making stiff joints more flexible.

- Turn you into a new, positive, optimistic, clear-eyed person feeling fitter and better than you have in years.

Wouldn't you be willing to give it a try?

Well, amazingly, there is such a therapy and it involves no pills or medication of any kind.

For five days you indulge in delicious salads, soups, and juices. The other two days you do *absolutely nothing*, needing only to go on breathing and drinking water.

We've devised a safe, at-home purification plan that combines two days of water fasting straddled on either side by several days of body cleansing foods. This sort of plan is the safest and most rapid way the body can relieve itself of arthritis aggravating foods and begin to use its energies for self-healing instead.

Although your doctor has probably never heard of cleansing therapy, and if he did he wouldn't believe in it, cleansing is widely used in natural healing.

A seven day purification plan is also the first part of the most reliable and accurate method of beginning GI tract healing and diagnosing food allergies. As the body cleanses, it becomes many times more sensitive to any food being tested. It also removes foods that are damaging your intestinal wall.

 Nature's Wonder Drug Ends Arthritis Pain

Fasting and cleansing provide rapid relief from most arthritis pain for several reasons. When food intake drops, so does immune response[28]—particularly the bothersome antigen-antibody complexes that settle in joints and cause trouble[33]. For a condition like rheumatoid arthritis where symptoms are provoked by overzealous body defenses, calmer immunity means less pain and swelling.

Not eating or only consuming easy-to-digest juices, broths, and fresh produce gives your gastrointestinal tract a break from refined foods and additives. This silences aching joints, particularly if poor digestion or other gastric complications are responsible for arthritic pains. Fasting and decreased consumption also decrease gut permeability making it harder for large, allergy prompting molecules to cross from the intestine into the bloodstream[34].

These dietary techniques abruptly cut off the allergenic foods that are causing arthritis symptoms. But when an allergenic food is reintroduced several days later, arthritis symptoms often reappear with renewed intensity. Because of this phenomenon, we are able to identify some foods that aggravate most forms of arthritis.

For example, Dr. Theron Randolph, an eminent Chicago allergist and one of the pioneers in allergy research, has reportedly fasted over 6,000 patients. The usual fast for his arthritis patients is reported to be 4–7 days. After arthritis pains cease, suspected foods are reintroduced one at a time. Allergenic foods often cause a swift flare-up of arthritis pain and symptoms.

A similar method is being used with overwhelming success at many small arthritis clinics and health resorts around the country. A consensus of their reports shows that after five days of not eating, 70 percent of arthritis sufferers temporarily lose all or much of the pain in their joints.

For instance, during 1980 a group of 15 patients with rheumatoid arthritis underwent a fast of 7–10 days at Linkoping Regional Hospital in Sweden. Ten others in a control group did not fast. After breaking their fasts, all 15 patients reported significant reductions in pain, swelling, and stiffness of joints, while none of the control group felt any better.

Interestingly, the study was made only to test the effects of fasting. Afterwards, the 15 fasters returned to their original diet and in 2–3 weeks all their previous arthritis symptoms returned.

Our program, of course, is to use a modified fast or cleansing diet to start intestinal recovery and identify the foods that are aggravating arthritis and to eliminate them from your diet. So, except while testing suspected allergy foods after the fast and cleansing period, you should—provided you stay faithfully with your eating program—experience considerable relief from rheumatoid arthritis symptoms. The only exception concerns gout and osteoarthritis where the necessity to bring your weight down to normal may prolong recovery time.

Seven days away from intolerant foods is considered sufficient for food allergy testing. Many of the success stories in this book mention five day fasts used by people to heal arthritis. However, all were conducted under the watchful eye of a physician. Do not embark on a water fast for more than two days without professional medical supervision.

 ## Dennis M. Obtains Permanent Relief from Rheumatoid Arthritis in Just Five Days

Dennis M. is typical of the thousands of arthritis sufferers that fasting has helped. We'll let him tell his story in his own words.

"For years, I'd suffered harrowing pain in my hands and knees. My hands were so stiff I could barely turn a doorknob. No drug gave me any benefit. But my doctor still went on giving me routine doses of cortisone.

"Finally, the constant pain became unbearable. I was ready to try anything. So I enrolled at a small natural foods spa in New Mexico.

"The chiropractor who ran it put me on an immediate water fast. For five whole days I ate nothing at all. But on the third morning, my pains ceased.

"Now, none of my friends will believe this, but by the last day of the fast, I was entirely free of pain. For the first time in years, all my pain had gone.

"I broke the fast with a meal of four oranges. This was the start of ten days of food testing in which I tested ten different foods— one each day. Each day I ate one test food like eggs, wheat, or chocolate. Three of the foods caused a severe flare-up. I learned that allergies to sugar, beef, and wheat were causing my arthritis.

"I was advised to drop these foods along with such obviously undesirable foods as white bread, fried foods, and all canned and processed items.

"Gradually, the stiffness and swelling in my joints disappeared. I stayed strictly with the diet. Within a year I was playing tennis again. And I've lived a completely normal life ever since."

 ## Tap Your Inner Wellsprings of Good Health

But, we hear you say, I couldn't possibly go two whole days without eating. I've never missed a meal in my life.

If that's the case, it may be why you have arthritis now. Unless you're obviously thin and underweight, almost all Americans tend to eat much more than they actually need.

Besides, food is a major contributor to arthritis. So what's wrong with giving your digestion a few days rest? Especially when those few days can end most arthritis pains forever.

The Three Categories of Fasting

This book may be your first introduction to fasting. That's why we offer a modified version—two days of water only, cushioned by another five days of simple nutritious meals and liquids. You'll gain considerable healing benefits, as well as eliminate allergy foods from your diet for seven whole days.

There are different levels to fasting, depending on your health, experience with fasting, and whether you are a do-it-yourselfer or under professional health care supervision. First timers wishing to water fast on their own, should limit their fast to one or two days. More experienced fasters, can go three or four days.

Longer fasts, those lasting from five days to a couple weeks, *should only be conducted with the assistance of a practitioner trained in fasting techniques.* Therapeutically, a lengthy fast can accomplish much, however, its intensity is too much for the layperson to handle alone.

Other Ways to Cleanse

If you absolutely cannot fast successfully—some people aren't built for fasting and do poorly on a water-only diet—you can try a restrictive diet. Instead of just drinking pure water, add herbal teas, homemade vegetable broth, and freshly prepared vegetable juices to your diet.

A juice fast is not a true fast because nutrients are consumed, hence the term restrictive diet. But it's the next best thing for those unable or unwilling to embark on a true water fast.

As with a water fast, consume as much broth and juice as desired. Avoid fruit juices at this point because they're high in fruit sugar which can send your blood sugar for a roller coaster ride and depress immunity. Dilute vegetable juices half and half with pure water.

While drinking juices and broths, versus just water, is more tolerable for some, there are disadvantages. A juice and broth diet requires preparation. The nutrients from broths and juices may also make you hungrier than you'd feel on water alone. You must be careful not to include suspected allergy foods and high allergenic foods (see Chapter 8).

Chapter 6 outlines detailed meal plans and recipes you can follow for a juice and broth only menu.

Who Should Not Undertake the Purifying Technique

A fast or cleanse will benefit just about everyone except pregnant women, nursing mothers, babies, or children, and anyone under essential medical care or with any of the following conditions:

Severe asthma, epilepsy, diabetes, heart disease or recent heart attack, advanced tuberculosis, cerebral disease, uncontrolled hypoglycemia, cancer, any blood disease, any active pulmonary disease, anemia, nephritis, peptic ulcers, eating disorders like anorexia nervosa and bulimia, or any form of mental illness. If you feel at all uncomfortable about fasting or cleansing, call your doctor.

This is not to imply that fasting or cleansing will not benefit most of these conditions. They frequently do. But complications could arise that call for professional supervision. If your doctor okays a fast with any of these ailments, fine! If not, you should fast only under the guidance of an experienced professional.

Again, if you are taking essential drugs for emergency treatment, or for maintenance purposes, you should have your doctor's permission before fasting. For drugs should not be taken during a fast or cleanse.

If you are taking non-essential drugs for arthritis or any other condition and there is no risk to life in stopping them, then you can safely drop them. Check with your doctor to be sure. He will probably advise you not to fast or cleanse. But the question to ask is whether there is any danger if you stop taking your medication for arthritis, or for any other condition. If the medication is simply to kill pain and reduce inflammation, there is seldom any risk in stopping it for a few days.

You can safely get rid of all non-prescription drugs before commencing to purify. Tranquilizers, sleeping pills, digestive aids or laxatives are all non-essential somewhat toxic drugs that will interfere with cleansing and food testing. Too, many people are allergic to aspirin.

Don't stop taking any drug or medication abruptly. Taper it off gradually for several days preceding the cleanse. This also applies to heavy coffee drinking. If cut off abruptly, coffee addiction can cause eight hours or more of throbbing headache the day following withdrawal. You can avoid this unpleasantness by phasing out coffee gradually and replacing it with herbal tea or a caffeine-free coffee substitute. Eliminate caffeinated soft drinks the same way.

Drug use should also be stopped during the several days of food testing that follow purification. If you cannot possibly stop all drugs, then go ahead while cutting down to the barest minimum. As you cleanse and pain disappears, try to reduce the dosage even more.

Finally, you should not undertake a fast or cleanse if you are at all emaciated, thin or underweight.

For anyone unable to fast or cleanse safely, alternatives are described in Chapter 9. They aren't quite as good for ending pain or for diagnosing allergies, but they are a satisfactory trade-off for anyone who should not fast. Also investigate the modified cleansing diet described in Chapter 6.

Seven Days May Be All You Need to End Arthritis Pain

Fasting is not starving. Fasting means that your body is feeding off its stored reserves of fat. Toxins have a proclivity for fat. As various toxins enter the body such as pesticide residues, drugs, stim- ulants, and chemical food additives, they end up in fat cells.

During a fast and to a lesser extent during a cleansing diet, fat cells are broken down to supply energy to fuel the body's metabo- lism. As they break down, fat cells release their stored-up toxins. The body then spews these toxins out through the kidneys, skin, lungs, and mouth.

As a result, the tongue acquires a whitish-yellow coat, the breath and skin become malodorous, the whites of the eyes may become discolored, and the urine turns brown. Fatigue, headaches, dizziness, and nausea may also arise during the fasting days. If any of these discomforts are disconcerting or ongoing, break the fast with cleansing foods. As long as these signs remain, it indicates that the body is still breaking down fat cells and is, therefore, still cleans- ing.

At the point where these signs disappear, fasting ends and starvation begins. When the breath and skin smell baby-fresh, the tongue is uncoated, the whites of the eyes are clear, and the urine is also clear, this indicates that the fast or cleanse must be broken.

Unless a person is already thin and emaciated, it is highly unlikely that the starvation point will be reached after fasting only two days. When you break your fast, you are still likely to display the coated tongue, brown urine, and malodorous breath and skin that indicate that detoxification is still incomplete.

Depending on the extent of surplus body weight, total detoxifi- cation for the average American may take 14–45 days or longer and require a weight loss of 10–45 pounds or more. Extremely obese peo- ple have fasted for months and have lost up to 200 pounds. Our mod- ified fast/cleanse gives you seven days of gentle body-wide house- cleaning, very different from these extreme examples.

A one-time, short two day water fast accompanied by another five days of mild cleansing will not undo years of poor eating. On the other hand, it's important that as a novice faster you feel comfortable and enjoy your first cleansing experience. That's why we suggest only two days on a water fast.

Think of fasting and cleansing in the same way you view exer- cise. Both are most beneficial to health when practiced regularly. Just as running 10 miles one day a year isn't going to do much to improve your well being (except maybe make you miserable and achy all over), fasting done intensely once in awhile isn't particularly helpful.

In this speedy obsessive driven world, it's easy to develop addictions to coffee, alcohol, sex, yes, and even fasting. Longer, harder fasts are not necessarily better for you. Take the gentle approach; become a frequent-flyer of fasting.

If the purification idea appeals to you, consider including regular, short fasts in your overall health plan. Some people fast one day a week. Others might enter a two-day water or juice fast once a month. Even a couple of days eating only fruits and vegetables and drinking wholesome broths and vegetable juices one to two days every month or two is a step in the right direction.

 An Easy Health Renewing Method Changes René N.'s Body Chemistry to That of a Teenager

René N. was 40 when rheumatoid arthritis first appeared in her left elbow. It soon spread to her left knee. Within months, René was unable to walk. Her doctor said there was no cure, and he prescribed 15 aspirin a day for life.

René's left knee swelled so badly that the synovial fluid had to be withdrawn by needle aspiration. Afterwards, she was placed on cortisone. But the only observable effect was new swelling in her right knee. Both knees became so badly swollen that René spent her days in a wheelchair.

Three years after the disease first appeared, René learned about fasting therapy from a friend who had just returned from a Nature Cure resort. René decided to begin a 5-day fast right away. (Don't try this at home.) Although her pain was too severe to cut out aspirin altogether, she reduced her intake during each day of the fast. When she broke the fast, she was taking only four aspirin per day, and at least half her pain had subsided.

René continued eating only natural foods as her friend had advised. She continued to show slow improvement. But then, René noticed that a flare-up would follow whenever she ate tomatoes, potatoes, peppers, or eggplant. Although little was known of food allergies at the time, René concluded that somehow these foods—all belonging to the nightshade family—were somehow responsible for her arthritis. She eliminated them altogether.

Within 15 days of cutting out nightshade family foods, the swelling subsided in both her knees and her elbow. Two weeks later, she got up out of her wheelchair and walked. Soon, she was climbing stairs and jumping, and she could even dance the Charleston.

In the ensuing 15 years, not a single flare-up has occurred. Today, at 60, René feels as fit and supple as she did at 18.

How the Seven Day Self Purification Technique Works

Within 24 hours of ceasing to eat or restricting food, profound biochemical changes begin deep within the body. Large amounts of blood and energy are released from the task of digestion and are directed into healing. Every organ and system in the body is rested and rejuvenated. As the kidneys free lymph and blood of toxic excesses, every cell in the body is gradually purified. Balance is restored to body chemistry and to each of the body's self-regulatory systems.

Besides feeding on its own fat cells, the body also consumes any cells and tissue that may be diseased, weak, aging, or dead. In this way, some of the damaged cells in arthritic joints may be replaced.

Let's not forget that all healing is self healing. When a surgeon sets a broken bone, he does not heal the bone. Only the body's own recuperative powers can rejoin the bone. Fasting and cleansing are wonderful ways to reduce disease and to initiate total health restoration.

While all this is going on, two events occur that are of paramount importance in arthritis recovery.

First, the body is relieved from the endless task of digesting refined foods. Instead, nutrients and energy can be rerouted to damaged tissues for repair.

Secondly, as allergenic food particles cease entering the bloodstream, they stop triggering the immune response. The huge swarms of surplus lymphocytes begin to disappear. The white blood cell count drops. And the lymphocytes cease their attack on arthritic joints in some people.

This is exactly how a fast and cleanse end the pain and other symptoms of many types of arthritis.

But unlike immunosuppressive drugs, which suppress lymphocyte activity only at the expense of lowering resistance, fasting and cleansing have no adverse side effects when carried out in a responsible fashion. In fact, some parts of the immune system become even more aggressive in protecting the body.

See and Feel Your Body's Healing Powers Destroy Arthritis

Little discomfort is experienced by the release of toxins into the bloodstream. But as foods are cut out or down, withdrawal symptoms frequently occur.

Any minor headache, dizziness, palpitation, nausea, vomiting, or possible skin eruption may be caused by withdrawal from food. Usually, food withdrawal symptoms appear as flu-like aches and discomfort during the first 1–2 days of a cleanse or fast.

Some people say they're addicted to certain foods, hence cravings for allergy foods. Theron Randolph, MD claims some people get hooked on foods much like others are to drugs. Other doctors disagree. Dr. Lisa Meserole of Seattle says, "Food allergies may manifest as addictive symptoms, due to inherited or individual biochemical idiosyncrasies, and create a type of craving. But eating a food repeatedly doesn't create an addiction."

Cleansing may enhance your yearning for favorite foods, but your uncomfortable symptoms, says Dr. Meserole, probably stem from withdrawal from stimulants (like coffee), medications, or other drugs. Low blood sugar and acidosis also create physical unease, as do waste elimination and healing.

So be prepared for some mild discomfort. With gout, acute flare-ups may occur as uric acid crystals are broken down and released into the bloodstream.

Try not to yield to any minor discomfort. *By the end of the fourth day most symptoms should have ceased.* From here on, your mind will become superbly clear, your nose will be free of congestion, and your senses of smell and taste will be unusually acute. Many people experience a calm euphoria free of all tension and anxiety. Depression and insomnia may vanish. By the seventh day, most people feel fitter and stronger than when the cleanse began.

However, if any symptom does give cause for concern during the two days of water, only you are perfectly free to break the fast at any time. Do so by eating a piece of apple or melon.

If vomiting or diarrhea persists, if your pulse rate is consistently high, if you have any prolonged weakness, headache, dizziness, or intestinal spasms, or any other alarming sign, don't hesitate to break the fast.

During the early stages of fasting and cleansing, many people do feel weak. So simply lie down and rest until you feel stronger.

Wonder Working Techniques That Overcome Hunger

You can ease hunger pangs during your two-day fast by sipping a cup of hot, pure water.

Acupressure offers another way to relieve hunger pangs. Locate the large lobe at the bottom of each ear. Just above it is another lobe that covers the eardrum. Pinch this lobe firmly between the finger and thumb. Do so on both ears simultaneously. Squeeze as hard as you can. Hold for 20 seconds, then release.

Now, immediately in front of this lobe (towards the eyes) locate a hollow. On each side of your head, press the hollow with the tip of your forefinger. Begin to press fairly hard. Hold the pressure to the slow count of 20, then release.

You can repeat this whole process two or three times if necessary. Your hunger pangs should cease for up to one hour, possibly more. You can repeat again whenever the pangs return.

Still another way to relieve the flu-like discomfort of food withdrawal is to experience it. Psychologists have discovered that whenever you experience something, whether pain, loneliness or boredom, it disappears. So place your awareness exactly where your hunger is located. Ask yourself where it is, what color it is, what shape it is, and how much water it could contain.

Keep your awareness focused exactly where your discomfort is located and keep answering the three above questions in rotation. In a very short time, your hunger pangs will disappear. If they return, repeat the process until the pangs disappear for good.

When and How to Begin

For employed people, the most convenient time to begin the purification plan is on Thursday morning. You can usually go through Friday without much discomfort. You can then relax at home over the weekend as you water fast. By Monday, you will begin eating again.

For your fast, choose a quiet, restful place free of disturbing noise and TV. Confine TV watching only to humorous shows and listening to soothing music. Don't strain your eyes with too much reading. Remember, rest is vital.

Avoid eating a huge meal the night before you cleanse. It's a good plan to cut down on meals for two or three days beforehand.

The first two days of your 7-day purification program should include lots of fresh fruits, raw, and lightly steamed vegetables. Avoid meats, dairy products, eggs, and any processed foods. Although cold water fish, seeds, nuts, beans, and legumes will eventually become part of your healthy eating plan, don't eat them during the purification program. Use olive and canola oils sparingly to season vegetables and grains. Lemon juice can be mixed with oils as a salad dressing. Grains will be added during the three days following your water fast.

Each day eat breakfast, lunch, and dinner, with three snacks spaced between meals and before bed. Remember, the object during cleansing days is to purify not go hungry.

Listen to Your Body's Instinctual Wisdom

If you have any misgivings about fasting, try an experimental fast. Start by skipping breakfast and noting how you feel. Actually experience hunger. A short while later, skip both breakfast and lunch. Study how you feel. Study your body's reactions. Learn how it is to feel hungry.

Try slightly underfeeding yourself for several days. At each meal, leave the table feeling slightly hungry. Learn how you react to hunger.

Some allergists believe that four days of cleansing is sufficient for testing most foods. But the majority prefer a 5-day abstinence from allergy provoking food.

True fasting and cleansing mean that besides water and/or cleansing foods you take in absolutely nothing but pure air and sunshine. That means no drugs, alcohol, vitamin or mineral supplements, mouthwash, toothpaste, chewing gum, chewing tobacco, candy, fruit juices, artificial beverages or stimulants of any kind. Avoid using deodorants, hairsprays, detergents, and commercial soaps and shampoos. It also means absolutely no smoking.

Barbara H. Comes Alive with Rejuvenated Health

Suppose, as in René N.'s case, pain is too severe for you to cut out painkilling drugs altogether. In that event, do as René did and reduce the dosage as steadily as conditions permit.

Consider the case of Barbara H., a 47-year-old secretary with polymyositis. This less common type of arthritis occurs when numerous muscles as well as joints become inflamed all over the body.

At first, aspirin relieved Barbara's pain. But the agony soon returned. Rasping pain radiated down the full length of both her arms and legs. Barbara constantly felt as though she had been poisoned. Soon, she was taking 18 aspirin a day.

Two years went by with no improvement. Then a friend told her about an arthritis clinic in a rural part of the state. Although Barbara did not believe in natural healing, as a last resort she decided to enroll.

"Within an hour of arriving, I was placed on a 5-day fast," Barbara said. "My pain was too severe to stop taking aspirin. So I continued with my regular 18 a day."

The aspirin didn't seem to make too much difference.

"After five days, my pain had been reduced by half—the first pain reduction in two years," Barbara went on. "I was overjoyed. I cut my aspirin down to only six a day."

Barbara was placed on a diet of fresh, natural foods and told to stay with them for life.

"Three weeks later, my pains had almost gone," she said. "And I'd discontinued aspirin altogether. I was able to walk and do housework with very little pain."

Gradually, her pains disappeared entirely and mobility returned. In six months, Barbara was completely back to normal. Now, 13 years later, she feels young and active and filled with so much energy that she dances and plays tennis several times a week.

Caring for Your Body as Arthritis Fades

During your 2-day fast, the only thing you may drink is pure water, preferably distilled or filtered, or else from a spring. Avoid well water or mineral water. Chlorinated or treated tap water is also undesirable. Drink whenever you feel thirsty, at least five cups daily. But it is not necessary to drink copious amounts of water.

During both cleansing and fasting days, brush your teeth several times daily with pure water and rinse out your mouth. This and gently scraping your tongue with a spoon or toothbrush will offset bad breathe and a coated tongue. Each day take a short tepid bath followed by a brisk rubdown with a stiff towel or loofah sponge to enhance toxin release—the skin is a major elimination organ.

Short sunbaths are beneficial but be careful not to burn. During summer, a 15-minute sunbath before 10 a.m. or after 3 p.m. is ample. Keep the body, and especially the feet, warm at all times especially at night as body temperature drops during a fast and cleanse. Try taking a hot water bottle to bed (don't use a heating pad or electric blanket).

Take a nap whenever you feel like it. Rest is imperative during a fast and cleanse to both facilitate tissue repair and conserve limited energy. Refrain from strenuous exercise or activities while fasting. A casual walk or light stretching are fine if so inclined, but no marathons. You may find that daytime resting and inactivity leaves you less sleepy at night—this is to be expected.

Keep notes on your body changes and how you feel. Enemas are not necessary for most people who fast and may in fact cause further discomfort. Constipation shouldn't be a concern; in fact while eating plenty of fresh fruits and vegetables should clear up any past constipation problems.

Breaking Your Fast

Break your 2-day fast on the morning of the fifth day. For example, if your last full meal is dinner on Wednesday evening, you would cleanse all day Thursday, Friday, then fast Saturday and Sunday. You would break the fast on Monday morning.

A short cleansing and fasting program such as this is not a long-term solution to a chronic condition like arthritis. But exiting even a two day fast incorrectly can undo all your hard work and perhaps create more problems than you started with. In other words, don't eat too much, too fast, too soon. As you re-enter the world of the eating remember to chew slowly and thoroughly, continue to limit quantities, eat foods at room temperature, and keep drinking liquids. Most importantly take time to enjoy your food.

You are purifying for many reasons—to cleanse and heal, as well as prepare for food allergy testing. So the foods you eat during cleansing days—two days before and three days after your fast—take thought. Read Chapter 6, describing the digestive diet used to repair your intestinal tract.

Then refer to Chapter 7 for instructions on investigating suspected allergy foods. Do not include these foods in your fast breaking menu or digestive diet. Select foods you seldom eat and are low on the allergenic totem pole (see Chapter 7).

Here's a suggested meal plan for the three cleansing days following your two day water fast. Continue to drink pure water, and consume vegetable broth and juices as desired.

DAY ONE

Breakfast: One piece of fruit (e.g., pear, 1/2 melon, grapes).

Lunch: One piece of fruit (different from breakfast).

Dinner: Vegetable soup (see recipe in Chapter 6).

DAY TWO

Breakfast: One or two pieces of fruit OR one cup of cooked whole grain, non-gluten cereal (e.g., rice or millet). No dairy.

Snack: One piece of fruit.

Lunch: a raw vegetable salad (see recipe in Chapter 6).

Snack: One cup of raw or steamed vegetables.

Dinner: Vegetable soup and well-cooked brown rice.

DAY THREE

Breakfast: Cooked whole grain, non-gluten cereal. No dairy.

Snack: One piece of fruit.

Lunch: Raw vegetable salad or steamed vegetables.

Snack: One piece of fruit.

Dinner: Whole grain, non-gluten cereal, steamed vegetables, and vegetable soup.

<u>DAY FOUR</u>

Digestive diet plan begins!

For those who prefer laboratory allergy tests (see Chapter 9), still follow the above suggestions then continue onto Chapter 6. Remember, fasting and cleansing are more than a diagnostic tool; they are also therapeutic. Skip Chapters 7 and 8 (though you may read them for information), and find a physician who will test you for foods best avoided.

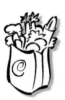

How Detoxifying the Body Helps All Forms of Arthritis

Should you cleanse for a mild form of arthritis such as bursitis or tendonitis? Provided you can do so without inconvenience, definitely yes. Although these nonarticular forms of arthritis usually begin with an injury, the injury does damage the body. And fasting and cleansing are healing therapies.

Even if you don't have any form of arthritis at all, it's best to eliminate any food allergies you can identify. For autoimmunity can cause other illnesses besides arthritis and not all food allergy symptoms are necessarily autoimmune related.

During seven days of purification, you may easily lose 2–5 pounds. Fluid is expelled and weight-loss is rapid. When you resume full eating, you will replace the fluid. But the fat you lost does not have to return. If you are overweight and especially if you have osteoarthritis or gout, a seven-day purification plan is a splendid way to launch a weight reducing program. As you progress to a diet of restorative foods, your weight will gradually reach its optimum level without further dieting. For more about losing weight, see Chapter 15.

It's Easy to Stop Smoking During Detoxification

You can use a cleanse as an easy way to stop smoking. Tobacco smoke is such a powerful poison that it always tests out as positive for *everyone* in *every* kind of allergy test.

That is why smoking is not permitted during a fast or cleansing diet. Even if it were, you would find smoking extremely unattractive on a nearly empty stomach. If you did get the urge to smoke during a cleanse and actually lit up, the result would be highly unsatisfying. People who light up again after a seven day purification report that their cigarettes taste like poison.

As a result, tobacco withdrawal symptoms simply mingle with fasting and cleansing symptoms.

Since it takes a week or less for complete physical withdrawal from tobacco addiction, when you complete your cleansing plan you will already have broken all physical dependence on nicotine. You will have absolutely no further physical need for cigarettes, pipes, or cigars.

Nicotine cravings, however, may haunt you for weeks, months, or even years. Adopting a wholesome natural diet void of addictive substances like caffeine and refined sugars will increase your success of maintaining a tobacco-free life.

So during purification, visualize yourself as starting out on an exciting new life as a non-smoker. Throw away all cigarettes, pipes or cigars, lighters, pouches or any other smoking paraphernalia.

Even when cleansing ends, you must not begin to smoke again while digestive healing and food allergy testing are in progress. That can occupy up to 17 additional days. So seize the opportunity and begin a new life free of both nicotine and arthritis! At no other point in life is it easier to quit as when you embark on a cleansing regimen.

Becoming a non-smoker is undoubtedly the greatest single step anyone can take towards improving health and adding years to his or her life. Because giving up smoking relieves the immune system of such a heavy overload of poisonous tar, nicotine, and other harmful chemicals not to mention disruptive free radical molecules, many people find that their arthritis improves significantly when they become non-smokers. Sometimes arthritis disappears altogether.

Special Healing Hints for Gout and Osteoarthritis

What if you cleanse seven full days and still have arthritis pains?

First, if you have gout, the pains are likely to continue or even to flare up during this time. This is because while cleansing, the body continues to break down uric acid crystals in the joints. The uric acid then enters the bloodstream causing a continuation of gout symptoms.

If you fasted for a long period, all uric acid deposits would be broken down and excreted. But that might take 2–3 weeks or even longer in an obese person—something we don't advocate you do on your own.

If gout persists, simply follow the directions laid out and go on with your planned digestive diet plan and food allergy tests. Low level pain may continue or diminish during the digestive diet week. But any allergenic food may produce a flare-up. Once you eliminate these allergy foods along with stressor foods that produce gout (see Chapter 11), the pain and symptoms of gout may gradually disappear.

The only other condition in which pain may continue after cleansing for one full week is osteoarthritis in which there is no autoimmune reaction. Excluding gout, most cases in which pain continues after cleansing 7 full days involve osteoarthritis caused primarily by physical wear and tear. In this case, the remedy is almost always to bring weight back down to normal so that the afflicted joints are relieved of the stress of carrying excess weight. Having come this far, though, a person with unrelieved osteoarthritis pain may just as well continue on with the planned food allergy tests and most definitely the steps that repair a leaky gut.

The GI tract healing plan which begins immediately when you finish cleansing is described in Chapter 6. Following that are instructions in Chapters 7, 8, and 9 on detecting sensitive foods—either on your own or with medical assistance.

Chapter **6**

The Digestive Diet
Plan That Helps
Arthritis Too

Arthritis isn't just sore joints. Natural medicine tells us that in order to eliminate disease and find optimal health, we must heal the entire body. Especially important in arthritic diseases are the gastrointestinal tract and liver. When these systems falter, symptoms amplify as food fragments, bacterial poisons, and other undesirables cross into the bloodstream. For some, this is how food allergies and autoimmunity begin.

Plugging Up a Leaky Gut

Now that you've cleansed for seven days, it's time to switch to a very basic, whole foods diet. This means lots of fresh vegetables and fruit, beans and legumes, non-gluten whole grains, some cold water fish, and a small amount of seeds. One week on this wholesome diet will further heal your bowel and other organs. Lucky for us the intestinal lining has the highest rate of cell turnover in the body and the greatest ability to self heal—given half a chance.

During your week of purification, you consumed fewer harmful substances and hopefully less allergy foods. When the gastrointestinal tract is saddled with toxins, the special immune cells that line your intestine, called secretory Immunoglobulin A (sIgA), get used up very quickly as they couple with incoming foreign antigens. Thus the digestive tract is left with fewer defenses. Seven days of easy eating allows your intestinal sIgA to replenish.

You also shunned alcohol and perhaps stopped taking your NSAID medicines, both substances that make a leaky gut leakier.

Before food particles enter general circulation, they are shuttled from the GI tract via special blood vessels to the liver. Once here they are detoxified and filtered. A seven-day cleansing diet reduces the amount of harmful compounds your liver must manage, allowing it to rest. Immune complexes that adhere to joints and initiate inflammation also decline during purification.

A Week of Healing Foods

Malnutrition makes a sieve-like gut even worse. So once initial cleansing is completed, it's time to step up to a more nutrient-rich week of basic foods to mend your insides. The antioxidant healers in fruits and vegetables lessen free radical insults to your gut. For one week you can eat all you want of the following foods:

Fresh raw fruits
Fresh vegetables (*raw or lightly steamed*)
Homemade vegetarian soup or broth
Freshly made vegetable juices
Dried beans (*soaked then cooked—time varies depending on the bean*)
Legumes (*as with beans*)
Brown rice
Quinoa
Amaranth
Millet
Raw, unsalted seeds
Cold water fish (*small servings—two to three times during the week*)

Pure water

Herbal teas

Herbal seasoning as desired

Cold-pressed canola or olive oil (*scant amount for salad dressings or seasoning*)

There are many excellent natural foods recipes and books on how to make delicious vegetable juices, broths, and other dishes using the above ingredients. To get you started, here are some simple, tasty recipes you can use either during your juice fast or as part of your digestive diet plan.

Dr. Medeiros' Healing Vegetable Juice

Dr. Faizi Medeiros from Norwich, Vermont, shares her favorite cleansing vegetable juice with us. Drink one cup daily during the purification program, digestive diet plan, or as a snack anytime.

Four carrots (greens removed)

One beet

Small handful of parsley

Three celery stalks (leaves removed)

1/4 inch sliced ginger root

You'll need a juicer to make this recipe. If you don't have one, try borrowing one to see if you'd like your own.

Bunch up parsley, push into juicer with carrots, followed by celery, ginger, and beet.

Invigorating Vegetarian Broth

Three quarts of water

Two onions, sliced

Four cloves of garlic, diced

One cup of red or green cabbage, sliced

Four carrots, diced

Four celery stalks, diced

One beet, diced

Handful of parsley, cut up

Any other vegetables you wish to add

After bringing water to a boil, add the vegetables and simmer for one to two hours. You can also use a slower cooker for four hours. Strain off the broth and drink as desired. If you want a tasty vegetarian soup, leave the vegetables in and serve.

Rainbow Vegetable Salad

Raw vegetable salads take very little preparation and a small amount of imagination. This is our favorite, but feel free to add what you enjoy.

One cup of torn romaine lettuce leaves

One half cup fresh spinach leaves

One half carrot, sliced

One half cup chopped broccoli

One quarter cup chopped jicama

A sprinkling of shredded beets

A sprinkling of shredded red cabbage

Two green onions, sliced

Two sprigs of parsley, cut up

Season, if desired, with lemon juice or a canola oil and balsamic vinegar dressing.

A Few Friendly Reminders

Ideally you will finish two weeks of nutritional cleansing and healing before testing for allergy foods. This means avoiding foods you suspect are causing troubles. Also include highly allergenic foods in your "Do Not Eat" list.

Fourteen days of such pure eating may also increase your reaction to allergy or intolerant foods. Be aware of this and eat only a modest portion of suspicious foods when testing. More about this in Chapter 7.

Excessive gas and flatulence can be a problem, particularly for anyone not accustomed to eating a high fiber and bean diet. Drink plenty of pure water and other fluids. Chew on or add fennel seeds to your recipes, a natural carminative or gas-reliever. The bitterness of fenugreek seeds aids digestive disturbances too. Also know that as your intestinal microbes change, bloating and gas will pass (no pun intended) within a few weeks. This is part of the healing.

For maximum GI healing, drink healing herbal teas like peppermint and chamomile. Take advantage of everyday kitchen spices that make for healthy digestion like caraway seeds, cardomon, coriander, ginger, thyme, and cayenne. See Chapter 14 for more suggestions on recovery foods for the digestion, in particular tips numbers 3, 6, 11, 13, 15, 16, and 20.

Foods That Stress the Digestive System

You are swapping your stressor diet of high saturated fat, protein, and simple carbohydrates for one jam packed with fiber and complex carbohydrates so your gut (and you) can find health again. It would seem that refined, cooked foods are easier to digest than the raw and whole. Actually the opposite is true.

Stressor foods, often packed with additives and preservatives, create intestinal changes which disrupt digestion and permit passage of oversized molecules—protein in particular—into the blood. This not only overwhelms a hardworking liver, but sends your immunity into a tizzy. When, during one study, rats were fed lots of junk food ladened with sugar and fat, their digestive enzymes fell[35]. Unlike fresh, raw foods, cooked refined foods have very little or no natural enzymes left. This places a greater demand on your body's digestive enzyme reservoir.

Eating on the run is another dinnertime sin. Chewing is the first step in digestion as food is smashed into tiny pieces; inhaling your dinner only makes it more difficult on your already harried gut (see Chapter 16). While it's certainly possible to wolf down a meal of brown rice and broccoli, natural whole foods with their rough, fiber-packed consistency demands more time and chewing before swallowing.

 ## Patricia B.'s Knees and Bloating Get Better

Patricia B. had always been very active, raising her three children, gardening, traveling with her husband, and running a bed and breakfast business in Victoria. Over the years, Patricia noticed stiffness developing in her knees. There was slight pain at times, but nothing she couldn't overcome with sheer willpower. For the most part, she carried on with her full schedule at age 54.

So it was a shock when one day her best friend, teary eyed, approached her and said: "Pat, you have to get help. You're walking like an old woman." Her husband was also concerned and called a local naturopathic doctor for advice.

After recording her lengthy medical history, the doctor suggested Patricia have X-rays taken of her knees; the results confirmed his suspicions of osteoarthritis. The doctor also noted Patricia's long history of gastric distress including bloating and stomach cramps after eating.

Patricia was immediately put on a cleansing diet. Within one week, the bloating and gastric pains went away. As Patricia learned how to incorporate natural foods into her diet and avoid wheat, her most prominent allergy food, her knees gradually loosened up. Within three months, her knees were limber and pain-free most of the time.

Since that time, she's added gentle, stretching exercises three times per week to her health regimen. The combination of natural eating and regular activity have given Patricia back the freedom to pursue the things she loves—without pain and frustration.

The Liver: Organ Extraordinaire

Tucked underneath the rib cage on the upper right side of the abdomen is your largest internal organ—the liver. The busy liver sticks to a hectic schedule of storing and filtering blood, producing bile for fat digestion, squirreling away vitamins and iron, as well as having a hand in almost every metabolic operation in the body. It should come as no surprise, then, that when such an influential organ gets sick or rundown, the rest of the body suffers. Sometimes this includes joints.

This major filtering system pulls poisons, drugs, chemicals, immune complexes, foreign antigens, and other undesirables from the bloodstream. Fortunately for us, a direct blood line runs between the GI tract and liver allowing the liver to discard most menacing material before it enters general circulation.

A well functioning liver uses its own brand of immune macrophages called Küpffer cells to snatch up bacteria trying to sneak into the body through the digestive tract. Cumbersome molecules and food pieces are also grabbed up and broken down into manageable bits by the Küpffers.

The Liver's Worst Enemies

As extraordinary as this organ is, being a liver in today's world is next to impossible. Pollution, food additives, drugs, cigarette smoke, alcohol, junk food, pesticides, and a sundry of other chemicals we meet everyday mean extra effort for your liver.

Your liver must sort through all these toxins while trying to keep you safe. Add to this load, waves of partly digested food particles, bacterial poisons, food additives, and other foreign antigens. How is a normal liver to keep up? When food antigens slip past the liver and spill into the bloodstream, immune complexes form—the stuff that gloms onto joints and causes inflammation. Poisonous endotoxins created by pathogenic bacteria also slip past the liver filter, adding to joint inflammation.

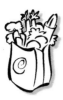

Using Fiber to Sweep the Intestines Clean

When we eat highly processed foods full of additives and void of nutrients, we miss out on intestinal cleaning fiber. Roughage and nutrients are discarded during food processing and refining; kind of like throwing out the baby instead of the bath water.

Fiber is the mostly undigestible stuff found in fresh fruits and vegetables, whole grains, and even beans and legumes. If it's not digested, why eat it, you might ask? Simple. Without fiber you become constipated and sicker in general. Low fiber intake is associated with diabetes, obesity, hemorrhoids, colon cancer, cavities, high blood pressure, and you guessed it, arthritis[36].

Eat food for roughage. Artificial fiber supplements and drinks tend to decrease mineral absorption.

A daily fiber infusion keeps your blood sugar even, decreases blood cholesterol, and helps fight cancer. And if you're trying to lose weight, there's nothing like a bowl of fiber packed vegetables and brown rice to fill you up.

Lots of fiber rich foods heal your ailing gut by increasing the release of digestive enzymes from the pancreas. More roughage means bulkier stools that pass faster and easier through the GI tract. The standard American diet contains a paltry 20 grams of daily fiber which means food takes at least two days to travel through the bowel.

People consuming a more basic, natural diet get 100 or more grams of fiber each day; their food passes through the body in a mere 30 hours or less.

Sluggish digestion increases your body's exposure to toxins—either ingested or created by bacteria. When you eat a healthful diet high in fiber, and low in sugar and fat, fiber binds to toxins in your intestinal tract and sweeps them from your body.

The intestine's good bugs use fiber to manufacture a short chain fatty acid called butyric acid as fuel for the gut and liver. Butyric acid also repairs and regenerates damaged cells in these areas. Some doctors supplement their patients directly with butyric acid pills. Nevertheless, increasing fiber is an important first step in your recovery plan. Too little roughage sends the bowel's microbe population into a tailspin as bad bugs overtake the good bugs. It's the bad bugs that make poisons like endotoxins, as well as launch other illnesses.

No More Bad Bugs!

Along with low fiber, saturated animal fats help create the "dysbiosis" or unsettling relationship between good and bad microorganisms in your gut. Animal fats also increase production of the inflammatory type prostaglandins that make your joints hot and red.

Normally there's a symbiotic or happy liaison between opposing microbe sides, each residing comfortably inside your intestine. The good bacteria, when in strong force, keep the delinquent germs at bay.

Excessive consumption of animal fats disrupts this comfortable association. Mary James, ND is director of Educational Services at Great Smokies Diagnostic Laboratory in Asheville, North Carolina, a lab specializing in the GI tract and digestive function. Meat and animal fats, says Dr. James, encourage *Bacteroides*, one brand of bacteria, to produce an enzyme that irritates the intestinal lining, promotes gastric inflammation, and leads to a leaky gut.

Garlic, green chlorophyll containing foods like spinach and broccoli, and various herbs like golden seal are natural antibiotics that decrease the pathogenic bugs in your digestive tract.

Reseeding Your Gut with Friendly Bacteria

Healthy foods makes your gastrointestinal tract liveable for its bacterial inhabitants. The next step in repairing your gastrointestinal tract is to replant some of the lost good bugs. An easy way to do this is by eating yogurt, fermented milk brimming with bacteria like *Lactobacillius acidophilus* and other friendly gut bacteria. A high fiber diet helps *Lactobacillius* grow more easily. Alcohol and antibiotics kill off this and other affable germs.

Lactobaccillius is but one of the 400 species living in the intestine, but is helpful in re-establishing a symbiotic gut population. Pills containing this and other friendly bugs, available at any health food store, can also be taken.

Reactivating Stomach Acid

There's no argument that stomach acid decreases with age which in turn impairs digestion and nutrient absorption. Dr. Robert Russell from the USDA's Human Nutrition Research Center on Aging at Tufts University in Boston says one-fifth of people over 60 with low stomach acid also suffer from bacterial overgrowth in the intestinal tract. This number doubles for those past 80[37].

Sipping on green tea or ginger root tea prior to a meal is a totally natural way of stimulating gastric acid for digestion. Bitter foods like lettuces and pungent leafy greens consumed in an apertif salad along with other raw vegetables get stomach juices flowing. See Chapter 14, recovery food tips numbers 6, 13, and 20.

Healing Your Liver Naturally

To complete the healing cycle, take care of your liver. Abandon as many chemicals, poisons, drugs, and other liver-damaging substances as you can. Eat organic foods, use non-toxic cleaners in your home, give up smoking and drinking (hopefully you did this during the purification plan), and ferret out every potentially hurtful chemical in your life. In other words, give your liver a break!

The 7-day purification plan and one-week digestive diet were the beginnings of healing your liver naturally. Without stressor or allergy foods to contend with, your liver can enjoy a two week furlough from filtering. Adding and sticking to restorative foods high in healing nutrients will further your liver's recovery.

Give your liver a rejuvenative boost by eating beets and dandelion greens with your meals. Prepare borscht or beet soup, steam beet roots and greens for supper, or grate raw beets on top of salads. Fresh dandelion greens are a wonderful wild food that gives salads an exotic appeal. Healing herbal teas containing milk thistle and dandelion root top off your liver rehabilitation schedule.

The next step is isolating food allergies with techniques coming up in Chapter 7.

Chapter 7

Allergy Foods That May Trigger Arthritic Disease

You can search for allergy foods on your own with a system called the elimination and challenge test. You've already eliminated suspected food allergens, now it's time to challenge your body to see if you react.

Some doctors swear by this method alleging it's the absolutely best way to test food intolerances. And in some ways that's true. You're in charge using this essentially free method, able to conduct it in privacy at home.

But like everything, it has its drawbacks. The elimination-challenge test requires perseverance, time, and patience from you. Because some food reactions are so subtle, it may be difficult to tell if any allergy is present or not. Other reactions will be obvious. Reactions that occur days or weeks after consuming an allergic food won't be picked up with this method.

Getting Started

Before cleansing—as far in advance as possible—start making a list of foods that you normally eat and to which you suspect you may be allergic. (Throughout this chapter and the remainder of this book, when we mention food it also implies beverages or drinks of all kinds.)

While many food allergens are found among health destroying stressor foods which are bad for everybody, we may also develop an allergy to a food such as citrus or lettuce that for most people is considered a desirable, health restoring food.

We're not quite sure why this is so. Some nutritionists claim that eating the same food every day creates an intolerance. But when you look at various cultures, each has its own favorite foods that its citizens eat regularly—Oriental countries like rice, corn is popular in Mexico. Perhaps poor diet, stress, and modern lifestyles that burden the intestine are to blame. Maybe the body reacts to pesticides and other chemicals swimming in food, not the food itself.

Whatever the reason, it's essential to restore bowel health and identify aggravating foods that may trigger an autoimmune reaction, like rheumatoid arthritis.

How to Identify a Food Allergy

Whenever a food to which we are allergic is omitted from a meal, we begin to experience vague discomfort. The meal seems incomplete and we may experience headaches, abdominal cramps, emotional stress, muscle aches, fatigue, or lack of energy and similar flu-like discomforts.

But food allergies are a complicated business. Many practitioners dislike the term food allergy, preferring intolerance or sensitivity, and wonder how many reactions to foods are true immune based allergies. Jonathan Brostoff and Stephen Challacombe, authors of the textbook *Food Allergy and Intolerance*, estimate true food allergies affect about 15 percent of all people[38].

It may take hours, days, or longer for an allergy food to cause a response, even after a week or more of abstinence. Even if when a delayed reaction occurs, the symptoms can be vague and hard to detect. Some food reactions occur only in the presence of another specific food.

Environment plays a huge role in shaping food allergies. Reactivity to food alters with the seasons, infection and even a woman's menstrual cycle. Hayfever and other airborne allergies enhance food reactions too.

Allergies, including to food, may crop up only when another activity or substance is putting additional stress on your body like exercise or poor nutrition. Even aspirin can cause enough stress to uncover a food reaction, as in aspirin-induced asthma. So if you're taking aspirin or other pain pills, kicking this habit may increase your tolerance to certain foods[38].

Answering the following questions can help uncover hidden food allergies. Answer each question by naming the foods concerned and remember that food includes beverages.

1. What food would you miss most if it were no longer available?
2. Must you eat any particular food the last thing at night in order to sleep?
3. Must you eat any specific food before you are able to face the day?
4. Must you eat any specific foods at lunch or during snack time?
5. Must you eat any specific food such as bread, potatoes, milk, eggs, or corn in some form at every meal?
6. Do you always stock up on certain specific foods because of a compulsive fear of running out?
7. Is any meal incomplete without a specific food?
8. Are you uncomfortable if you miss a meal, or are late for a meal, containing certain foods?
9. Would the discomfort be relieved if you ate the food?
10. Does eating a certain food always seem to be followed by a flare-up of arthritis?
11. Does eating a large quantity of any food always seem to be followed by a flare-up of arthritis symptoms?
12. Does eating any food invariably cause indigestion, heartburn, gas, or gastrointestinal trouble of any sort?
13. Do you find eating certain food combinations cause reactions, while eating these foods alone do not? (See pages 198–199)
14. Do you only react to a particular food after taking certain medication?
15. Does exercise or exertion bring on food reactions?

16. Do your food reactions change from season to season?

17. Are your food allergies worse during a cold, flu, or other illness or infection?

18. For women: Do you react to foods more during certain times of the month?

Joan B.'s Arthritis Disappears When She Unmasks Her Hidden Food Allergies

How well can the preceding questions help you identify arthritis causing foods?

Similar self-inquiry certainly helped Joan B. who, for four years, had suffered agonizing pains from rheumatoid arthritis in her hands and left knee. Her doctor had tried a whole arsenal of drugs on her without success. But let Joan tell her own story.

"All the drugs did was to worsen the abdominal cramps and diarrhea I'd been suffering from for years. Together with the arthritis, it was all so bad I had to give up my typing job to stay home and rest.

"Then in 1978 I read in a medical journal that allergy to common foods was suspected as the cause of rheumatoid arthritis. I knew nothing of fasting or food testing at the time. But I decided to phase out my drugs and to go ahead and do something about my arthritis on my own.

"So I analyzed my eating habits. I strongly suspected I was reacting to bread, sugar, tomatoes, hamburger, and coffee. I went right ahead and just cut out those foods completely.

"I did feel slightly uncomfortable for a few days without my favorite foods. But after a week, the arthritis began to improve, quite noticeably. And for the first time in years, my digestive pains cleared up completely.

"I still had low level arthritis pain and stiffness. But I was really elated with my success. So I consulted an MD, who specialized in allergies. He congratulated me and said I had probably uncovered a masked allergy to all of the foods I suspected.

"Just to be sure, though, he put me on a purifying fast, then had me eat test meals of wheat, rye, yeast, sugar, tomatoes, hamburger, and coffee.

"I tested allergy positive to wheat, sugar, hamburger, and coffee. But I'm still able to eat rye, yeast, and tomatoes. I'd never have known this without fasting and food testing. I'd have gone on avoiding rye, yeast, and tomatoes unnecessarily."

Although some deformity remains, Joan has recovered much of the mobility in her hands and knee. She still cannot type, but loves her new job as a receptionist. Today she leads an active and completely normal life.

Why We Don't Need to Challenge Stressor Foods

As you read in Chapters 3 and 5, the body develops gastric problems and possibly food allergies as a result of marginal nutrition. People who enjoy optimal nutrition have healthier guts and tend to develop fewer food sensitivities; arthritis is also less of a problem. By contrast, many with arthritis suffer from a serious nutritional deficiency.

To recover from arthritis, we must cut out all stressor foods—those health destroying foods that nutritionally deplete the body and create physical stress—and replace these bad foods with health-building restorative foods.

But it takes time to rebuild a run down body and to restore the damage done by years of wrong eating. Which is why our second goal after repairing the gut and liver is to identify and phase out those allergenic foods that may trigger rheumatoid arthritis.

Nonetheless, if you hope to become permanently free of arthritis, you should put recovery Steps 1 and 4 into effect immediately. That is, you should cut out all stressor foods and replace them with restorative foods.

You'll find a description of stressor foods in Chapter 11. But here is a brief outline:

FAT: hydrogenated vegetable oils and margarine; saturated fats—butter, lard, all fatty meats.

ALCOHOL: all liquor, beer, and wine.

CAFFEINE: coffee, black tea, chocolate, cocoa, some soft drinks.

REFINED CARBOHYDRATES: sugar, white flour, white rice, and all refined flours and cereals.

SWEETENERS: aspartame, saccharine, or any other artificial sweetener. Any food or drink containing sugar, fructose, or any sweetener listed here.

PROCESSED FOODS: any packaged, processed, convenience, canned, precooked, manufactured, prepared, artificial, substitute or fast food. Includes sausages, luncheon meats, and smoked meats; also all processed baked goods.

ADDITIVES, CHEMICALS: any food containing artificial chemicals or additives, including MSG.

Any food product containing one or more stressor foods must be considered equally taboo. The list extends to practically every food carried on supermarket shelves.

Now since you will be avoiding these foods, it is superfluous to spend time testing any Stressor Food.

 Never Say Never Again

We hate to say never eat a particular food ever again. For one, such strict dietary demands backfire on most people. We've learned this painful lesson with weight loss diets. People who shun certain foods in the name of thinner bodies often feel deprived and end up gorging on the very fattening foods they avoided in the first place.

Secondly, you must decide how many changes you want to make in order to get well. Some people aren't willing to make the enormous dietary leap from their standard fare to a very natural, whole foods, no chocolate chip cookies-ever-again diet.

So, here's the deal. Try two weeks of cleansing, see how you feel. Test foods you think are causing reactions and avoid them. THEN decide what foods are worth avoiding forever, and what ones aren't.

It's enough for some people to settle for a mere decrease in pain by following only a few of our guidelines.

Only Basic Foods Should Be Tested

A basic food is something like wheat, sugar, soybeans, coffee, milk, or corn which cannot be broken down into any component foods. For instance, most breads are not basic foods. They may contain wheat, rye, sugar, yeast, soy oil, shortening, and other basic foods. Only unleavened bread made of flour and water and nothing else is considered a basic food.

Thus any item such as lasagna, mayonnaise, pancakes, fried foods, soft drinks or ice cream that contains more than a single basic food must be tested by separately challenging each ingredient. If you suspect hamburgers, for instance, your sensitivity may be to the wheat, sugar, or yeast in the roll or to the meat itself. With bread, you may be sensitive only to yeast and not to any of the other ingredients. With fried foods, you may be allergic to the food itself or to the fat it is fried in.

Therefore only basic foods should be tested. And each basic food must be challenged separately.

(If for some special reason you do wish to test a non-basic food such as commercial bread or a stressor food like sugar or white rice, the test procedure is the same as for basic foods. However, you will not be able to identify exactly which ingredient of bread is the real culprit. And since stressor foods create the condition of nutritional stress which precedes arthritic disease, you should not be eating these health wrecking foods at all.)

Making Your Arthritis Food List

The next step is to break down your list into basic foods. Head your list with the basic foods you suspect you react to, you crave most of, eat most often, and eat the largest amounts of. Then add the remainder in decreasing order. (*These are also stressor foods.)

Wheat	Pork and bacon
Milk and cheese	Chicken
Eggs	Lamb
*Sugar	Oats
Beef	Brown rice
*Coffee	Soybeans and soy products
*Chocolate	Honey
Veal	Peanuts
Tongue	Tomatoes
Canned tuna fish	Lettuce
Oranges	

The Foods That Aggravate Arthritis

To give you a better idea of foods to which you may have a hidden allergy, here are lists of the most common, fairly common, and rare foods that may exacerbate rheumatoid arthritis.

Statistically you are most likely to have an allergy to such foods as sugar, wheat, milk, corn, soy, caffeine, eggs, and chocolate. But every person has a unique body chemistry. You may find you have no sensitivity at all to any of the most common allergy foods but a reaction to one or more foods in the "fairly common" or "rare" groups.

While you'll want to eliminate the most common allergens during your two weeks of cleansing, the rare allergen list gives you foods you can eat comfortably (unless they belong on your personal avoidance list).

Most Common Allergens

Drugs

Tobacco smoke

*Alcohol (*wine, beer, hard liquor*)

Buckwheat

*Chocolate

Citrus fruits (*oranges, lemons, limes, grapefruit*)

*Coffee and black tea

Coconut

Corn (*also derivatives like corn syrup*)

Cow's milk (*and dairy products like cottage cheese and butter*)

Eggs

Fish—all types

*MSG

Nuts (*including nut oils*)

Peanuts and peanut butter

Pineapple

Pork (*ham, bacon*)

*Soft drinks

Soy (*a common additive*)

*Sugar and candy

Strawberries

Tomatoes

Vinegar

Wheat (*and its products including bread*)

Yeast (*bakers and brewers*)

Fairly Common Allergens

Apples

Chicken

Cucumber

Green beans

Green and red peppers

Mushrooms

Onion

Potatoes

Spinach

Rare Allergens

Apricots

Artichokes

Asparagus

Barley

Broccoli

Carrots

Grapes

Honey

Lamb and mutton

Lettuce

Oats

Peaches

Pears

Raisins

Rice

Rye

Sweet potatoes

Usually, if you have a sensitivity to soy, wheat, rye, corn, or similar foods from which other products are made, you will be sensitive to these other food products also. But with milk, this is not always true. People with a sensitivity to milk, cream, and hard cheese may not be sensitive to cottage cheese or yogurt. So it might be necessary to test milk products separately.

While homogenized milk can be allergenic, raw milk and all raw milk products are often well tolerated. Cow's milk is the principal culprit. Goat's milk produces allergies less often although someone who is allergic reacts to cow's milk can also react to goat's milk.

You probably noticed that peanuts and nuts are listed separately; that's because peanuts are actually legumes, not nuts. We'll be singing praises for fish later, but since fish can cause reactions in some individuals, leave them off your menu until allergy testing time.

One more thing, gluten, a protein found in most grains including wheat, barley, and oats, can cause problems. See Chapter 8 for more details.

A Severe Case of Arthritis Ends When Allergy Foods are Dropped

Can less common forms of arthritis be helped by eliminating allergenic foods?

Richard A., a 28-year-old accountant, was diagnosed by X-rays as having ankylosing spondylitis. Since the onset of his disease, Richard had become a great believer in natural healing and was well acquainted with cleansing and nutritional therapy. Fortunately, Richard's doctor was also personally interested in allergy and nutritional therapy and he agreed to cooperate in reversing Richard's arthritis without drugs.

Because one person in four with ankylosing spondylitis is afflicted with inflammation of the eyes, Richard's doctor recommended maintaining minimum medication to prevent eye inflammation. The doctor gave Richard his blessing and took him off all aspirin and other non-essential drugs.

Richard immediately began a 7-day cleansing diet. The pain and inflammation in his lower spine and legs began to decrease. But when he completed the week, low level back pain still smoldered on. His doctor said they were caused by the maintenance drugs. Even so, Richard felt sure he could recognize a flare-up caused by any food sensitivity.

Richard's doctor instructed him to test one new food each day. The foods, of course, were common allergens. Both sugar and wheat produced severe pain in his sacroiliac. Milk brought pain and stiffness in his lower back and legs. Beef left him feeling tired and his spine poker stiff.

These foods were dropped immediately and were replaced with whole, fresh natural foods and produce. Richard's ankylosing spondylitis didn't disappear overnight. But over the next six months he gradually became so free of arthritis symptoms that his doctor took him off all medication.

It's too early to tell whether Richard's remission is permanent. But his back is neither rigid nor fused in a curve—the usual end results of ankylosing spondylitis—and he is still free of all arthritis symptoms.

The Foods You Challenge Must Have Been Eaten Recently

When your list of suspected basic foods is complete, check to be sure that you've actually eaten all of these at least once or twice during the five days preceding your fast.

This is because when you stop eating a non-tolerated food, your sensitivity to it increases sharply for the next several days. If you eat an allergenic food after having abstained from it for, say, three or four days, it will produce a sharply magnified reaction.

But after a week or more has gone by without eating the food, the immune system often begins to lose antibodies to it. After abstaining from a food for several weeks, that food may no longer test out as allergenic or its symptom will be delayed or vague.

For a non-tolerated food to show an allergenic response, it should be eaten at least once or twice in the five days preceding your fast. (The same applies when using any alternative method of food testing.)

Fixed food allergies are much easier to detect. Eating these foods creates a very definite reaction, whether you've consumed them recently or not. Fixed allergies can also be more dangerous. If you know you have a strong allergic response to a particular food, *do not test it at home on your own. Test fixed food allergies only with your doctor's help using the elimination-challenge technique or laboratory allergy tests.*

The Self Purification Technique
Magnifies Food Sensitivity

During the first few days after two weeks of cleansing, the allergic foods you eat may magnify arthritis symptoms. If they are allergenic, the first few foods you eat may produce symptoms of arthritis or other discomfort in just a few hours or less. But the power of this reaction gradually diminishes. Thus we suggest testing foods for no longer than 10 days following the end of your fast.

We Lose Sensitivity to Foods When We
Stop Eating Them

If you abstain from a non-tolerated food while eating normally, you would probably lose most sensitivity to that food within two weeks or so.

But the sensitivity quickly returns when you begin to eat the food regularly again. For example, if you abstained from a food for six weeks, then ate it once, you would probably experience no reaction. But that single exposure is sufficient for your immune system to build fresh antibodies. If you then begin eating that food every day, or every second or third day, the original sensitivity rapidly returns.

Even after taking these precautions, some food reactions will be vague, delayed for days or require additional circumstances to set them off. While you won't identify these foods, you will pick up others thus solving at least part of your arthritis food puzzle.

We Can Often Eat Allergy Foods Again If We Heal Our Gut and Add Variety to Our Diet

In many cases, taking care of a damaged digestive tract corrects food intolerances. This is especially true for hidden allergies and anyone cursed by a multitude of sensitivities.

As you replace stressor foods with restorative foods, and your body begins to regain its health, you probably can begin eating some of your favorite allergy foods again.

For example, if after abstaining for six-to-eight weeks or more, you begin to eat a non-tolerated food only at well-spaced-out intervals, the original sensitivity often does not build up to its former intensity. A properly functioning intestine and happy liver also discourage large food particles from entering your bloodstream and annoying your immune system. By adding variety to your diet and spacing out meals of previously allergenic foods, you may very well be able to continue to enjoy them.

Foods that you can eat again on a rotating basis after a period of abstinence are known as *cyclical* allergens. Very often these kind of reactions are tied to a leaky gut, especially in a person with no history of allergies—food or otherwise.

However, some foods *always* set off a reaction. Regardless how long you abstain or how little you eat, every time you eat that food a flare-up follows. Such foods are called *fixed* reaction allergens and their antibodies seem to remain in the bloodstream indefinitely. They show up in allergic-type people. When, after an abstinence, the food is eaten again, a flare-up of arthritis symptoms may soon follow.

Leonard K.'s Mysterious Weekend Arthritis

Flare-ups are often set off when a person who has changed to a health restoring diet lapses and goes on an eating binge of allergenic or refined foods. Even though only one of the foods may be a fixed reaction allergen, this is sufficient to trigger a painful flare-up of arthritis pain and swelling.

Leonard K., a stockbroker, has a flare-up of rheumatoid arthritis regularly every Sunday and Monday. The pain and inflammation gradually die away by the following Friday.

About 15 years ago, Leonard underwent a cleanse and food tests. He carefully dropped all allergy-positive foods from his diet along with most stressor foods. Within a few weeks, the rheumatoid arthritis pain in his ankles and knees subsided and he seemed well on the way to recovery.

Then something went wrong. Every weekend, Leonard's pain and inflammation returned. And though it gradually diminished during the week, it never had a chance to really get better. Because the following weekend, Leonard experienced still another flare-up.

"You're eating something you shouldn't," a friend told him.

"Absolutely not," Leonard said, "come to dinner Saturday night and see."

Leonard's statement was literally true. But in nutritional therapy, food means everything we take into our mouths including smoke, drugs, and beverages.

During the evening, Leonard sipped his way through at least four generous tumblers of bourbon on the rocks.

"There's your trouble" his friend said. "Alcohol is a fixed reaction allergen. Cut out the liquor and your arthritis will disappear."

"I've decided not to," Leonard said. "The comfort I get from drinking on weekend nights is greater than the discomfort of arthritis during the week."

The moral here is that learning which foods cause your arthritis does not stop the disease. To overcome arthritis you have to cut these foods and drinks out of your diet—and keep them out. The decision is yours.

The Challenge: Testing One Food at a Time

Continue consuming meals based on the digestive diet plan. Begin the challenge by eating one serving of your first allergy food with breakfast. Don't eat your tested food for the rest of the day.

Next day, you repeat the same thing with the next food to be tested. Since you can continue testing for 10 days after the two week cleanse, this allows you to test 10 different foods.

Now, 10 basic foods may not seem like many. But, remember, you don't need to test any stressor foods.

Let's return for a moment to the list of typical suspect foods given earlier. Of these 21 foods, 3 carried an asterisk showing they are stressor foods and need not be tested. Hence only 18 foods required testing. And as lists go, this one is unusually long.

If you do have more than 10 foods to test, here's how to handle it. Test the 10 foods that you suspect most at the rate of one per day. Then check out the remainder with the alternative tests described in Chapter 9.

Using our same list of suspect foods, here's how your 10 day test meal schedule might look:

Monday: oranges	Saturday: lamb
Tuesday: chicken	Sunday: brown rice
Wednesday: wheat	Monday: soybeans and soy products
Thursday: veal	Tuesday: tomatoes
Friday: oats	Wednesday: peanuts/peanut butter

If other foods continue to cause problems, you can test them later by an alternative method.

Drugs May Confuse Test Results

Throughout the test period, except when testing a beverage, drink only pure water. Chewing gum is forbidden as are smoking, alcohol, and drugs.

If you do smoke, drink alcohol, or take a drug, it will invariably provoke a reaction and test out as allergenic. Should you be unable to complete the cleanse and test period without foregoing aspirin or a prescription drug, recognize that the drug will invoke a continual reaction. Any other allergenic reaction will be superimposed upon it.

Knowing this, you may still be able to identify any flare-up caused by the allergenic foods you are testing. But drugs only confuse the task of identifying food allergens. If at all possible, you should drop all non-essential drugs before commencing the cleanse.

A Simple Food Test Helps Roberta A. End Her Arthritis

Roberta A., a 38-year-old waitress, had rheumatoid arthritis in her left knee for 18 months. Besides the routine 15 aspirin per day and occasional steroid injections, her doctor advised wearing a rubber stocking over her knee. But it didn't really help. After one particularly painful flare-up, Roberta had to give up her job. Unable to climb stairs any longer, she slept on the living room sofa. Even then, the pain was so severe she could sleep only when tranquilized.

A friend who worked in a health food store told Roberta about research that had identified food allergies as one cause of rheumatoid arthritis.

With her friend's help, Roberta reviewed her diet and found that each day she ate 10 thick slices of whole wheat bread spread with peanut butter plus six cups of strong coffee, as well as eggs, beef, cheese, and a large helping of spaghetti made from wheat. On Roberta's list of suspect foods were wheat, coffee, yeast, peanuts, eggs, beef, and cheese.

Under her friend's direction, Roberta was to cleanse for four days after which she was to eat one suspect food each day for the following seven days.

As she finished her cleansing diet on the fifth morning, Roberta realized that much of the pain had disappeared from her knee. But after her first two meals of cooked wheat, she was back on the sofa with one of the worst flare-ups she had ever experienced. Of the other foods, only coffee, beef, and cheese precipitated arthritis symptoms.

Roberta dropped these four culprit foods and replaced them with health building foods suggested by her friend. In 14 days, the pain and swelling in her knee had almost disappeared. A month later she was walking freely. In the 12 months since, she has worked steadily at her job. And only once, when she strayed from her diet, did her pains briefly return.

(Note: One of Roberta's foods, coffee, was a stressor food which we would not need to test.)

How Test Foods Should Be Prepared

Each food should be prepared the way you normally eat it either cooked or raw. If you eat it both ways, eat half the meal cooked, half raw. Buy foods from the same sources as usual. If you normally buy lettuce in the supermarket, don't get organically grown lettuce for the test. If you normally eat a certain grade of meat, test that grade not another grade that may have more or less fat. If you normally eat apples with the skins on, don't peel them for the test. You may be reacting to pesticide residues on the skin.

Foods such as honey, yeast, or spices cannot form a regular meal. Yet each must be tested singly like any other food and allotted the same period of time for a reaction to show up. Here is how certain foods should be tested.

BAKER'S YEAST: stir one tablespoon of commercial baker's yeast into a glass of pure, chlorine-free water and drink.

BREWER'S YEAST: stir one tablespoon of brewer's yeast into a glass of pure, chlorine-free water and drink.

OATS: the meal should consist of plain, dry puffed oats and/or plain oatmeal prepared in pure, unchlorinated water—depending on how you normally eat oats.

RYE: boil then simmer some plain rye in a double cooker or over a slow burner until tender. Use only pure, unchlorinated water. You may also eat rye crackers made without yeast or sugar.

WHEAT: cook some plain wheat berries or cracked wheat in a double cooker or over a slow burner until done. Use only pure, unchlorinated water. Alternatively, make some chapatis (flat bread) of whole wheat flour and pure water. Sometimes matzoh is also made of pure wheat.

HONEY: stir three tablespoons of honey into a glass of warm, pure water and drink. Similar amounts of any other naturally-occurring sweetener may be tested in the same manner.

WATER: pure water is never allergenic. But tap water treated with large amounts of chlorine, fluoride, water-softening chemicals, or other additives may very well be. Well water may also contain heavy pesticide or fertilizer residues. Mineral-rich spa water can also be allergenic. Reserve a full meal period for testing suspected water and drink as much as you comfortably can. You can drink it warm if you prefer.

Bear in mind that any food which you normally prepare by mixing with a considerable volume of water, such as oatmeal or grits, may not itself be allergenic. Your allergy may be to the treated water.

Because you're eating varied and full meals through the challenge, you should feel full and satisfied. However, don't add salt, butter, pepper, or any kind of condiment or seasoning to your test food. If you are testing potatoes, your meal should consist only of baked, boiled, or steamed potatoes. Never fry or use any method of preparation that would introduce another food.

Chapter 8

How to Identify

Allergy Foods

After eating a test food, what reactions should you expect and when?

First, your challenge meals may reveal the existence of allergens that cause ailments or symptoms other than arthritis, such as migraine headaches. If this happens, you will naturally want to drop that food also even though it doesn't aggravate arthritis. Any food that produces dizziness, nausea, weakness, fatigue, fever, or headache should be suspected as a possible cause of any other chronic ailment you might have. These symptoms can appear quite soon after eating the culprit food, sometimes within an hour.

Throughout your days of food testing, keep careful notes. Record the exact time of each meal and the times at which any symptoms appear.

Pinpointing the Foods That Aggravate Arthritis

How long does it take for symptoms to appear? After eating an arthritis aggravating food, it usually takes 6–18 hours for arthritis symptoms and joint pains to appear. But during the first few days following the cleansing diet—when sensitivity is magnified—reactions may be even swifter. We have seen joint pains appear as rapidly as three hours after a test meal.

Of course food reactions can take days to show up. And you never know if other factors or foods need to be present in order to tip off an allergenic response. However, you can be reasonably sure that a food is at the root of your problem when reactions to it are strong and swift.

You will recognize these drastic food reactions because, at latest, symptoms will appear first thing the following morning. Harking back to the sample test schedule in Chapter 7, if you woke up the first Wednesday with stiff and painful joints, you can be reasonably sure it was caused by the chicken you tested the previous day. (See page 124.)

Another example: Let's say that on the Saturday you experience a flare-up about 9 p.m. It was probably caused by the lamb you had been eating all day.

Again, if a flare-up occurred at noon on the second Tuesday while you were eating tomatoes, and continued at full strength for the remainder of the day while you continued with your tomato meals, the culprit food is almost certain to be tomatoes, the tomatoes you have been eating since breakfast.

There is, of course, a slight possibility it might have been caused by Monday night's soybean dinner, since you ate this dinner less than 18 hours previously. You should record this overlapping possibility in your notebook. Also jot down other possible aggravating factors like a bad night's sleep, exercise, or a particularly stressful day.

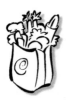 ## A Simple Way to Identify Culprit Foods

Where there is any overlapping doubt as to exactly which of two foods may be aggravating arthritis, reading and writing tests can often help identify the non-tolerated food. Although reading and writing is affected only by the more severe allergens, these tests are often useful in confirming which of two or more suspect foods is the exact one to which you have a sensitivity.

Reading and writing tests must be made after each test meal. About 30 minutes after eating a test meal, begin to read a magazine. If the type appears blurred or you see double, this is a strong indication that the food you recently ate is allergenic.

For confirmation, write your name several times followed by a few sentences in longhand and two rows of figures. Then print a couple of sentences. If your writing tends to become a scrawl, or is barely legible, or if occasional letters or figures are omitted or written backwards, this is a strong indication that your last meal was allergenic.

These reading and writing checks must be made at intervals of 30 minutes for four hours following each test meal. If you get a reaction, the food may not necessarily be causing the arthritis. But you very probably have a strong sensitivity to it.

Reading and writing tests are now widely used in allergy clinics to confirm food sensitivities. While testing foods for arthritis, they helped Myrtle L. uncover two migraine causing food allergens that she would otherwise have overlooked completely.

Simple Food Tests Help Myrtle L. End the Pain of Both Arthritis and Migraine

For years, Myrtle L., a computer programmer, was plagued with severe migraine attacks. Soon after her 39th birthday, pain and swelling appeared in Myrtle's wrists and soon spread to her elbows, knees, and neck. After tests confirmed it was rheumatoid arthritis, a friend—who had already recovered from arthritis through nutritional therapy—suggested that Myrtle consult an allergist.

When the allergist discovered that Myrtle was a heavy eater of devitalized foods, he placed her on a five day fast. Most of her joint pains disappeared during the five foodless days. Myrtle then began to test a suspected allergy food at the rate of one per day.

At intervals of 30 minutes after each meal, she was instructed to read a magazine and to write several sentences in longhand and print. An hour after eating a plateful of cooked wheat, Myrtle could hardly read the magazine—the print was so blurred. And her usual firm, round handwriting became a barely legible scrawl. Several hours later, she experienced severe pain in her wrists and knees.

Myrtle noticed the same blurred vision and scrawled handwriting after meals of cheese and chocolate. But only the cheese produced arthritis pains. On the day following the chocolate tests, she experienced a severe attack of migraine headache.

After dropping all three foods, Myrtle's arthritis symptoms gradually disappeared, and her migraine attacks became increasingly rare.

How to Use the Same Techniques That Successful Arthritis Clinics Employ

The cleansing and food testing methods described here are virtually identical with those being used in the most successful and most expensive allergy clinics that help thousands of people with rheumatoid arthritis every year. By following instructions carefully, you can achieve similar results in your own home without spending a penny.

If, after a flare-up occurs, pain and stiffness have not decreased by at least 50 percent, postpone testing the next food.

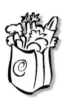

How to Interpret Signs of Food Sensitivity

During food tests, flare-up symptoms may begin to die down in a few hours after you stop eating the culprit food. Usually, pain and stiffness caused by a previous day's flare-up will decrease overnight.

However, before continuing with your tests, wait for symptoms to diminish to where you can readily recognize another flare-up if it occurs. Meanwhile, go on eating meals based on your digestive diet plan. Often you will not have to wait more than 24 hours before symptoms have abated to where you can continue testing. As soon as symptoms have diminished appreciably, proceed with food testing.

Should you experience one or two prolonged flare-ups, you may not have sufficient time to test all 10 suspect foods in the 10 days at your disposal. In this event, you can test the remainder with the alternative techniques described in Chapter 9.

Provided you test foods in approximately the order you suspect them, two or three flare-ups should serve to identify the most potent allergens that are aggravating your arthritic disease.

Food Testing Helps Bob W. Phase Out Rheumatoid Arthritis

Forty-eight year old Bob W. had rheumatoid arthritis for three years. His doctor prescribed drugs that suppressed the pain and swelling. But the side effects caused constant discomfort. Finally, Bob consulted a new doctor well versed in nutrition. Bob was told to drop all stressor foods. Despite this, Bob continued to experience bouts of intense pain in his knees and wrists.

His doctor sent Bob to a small arthritis clinic in the Southwest for cleansing and food testing. Bob was delighted when, after five days of cleansing, his pains disappeared. He then began to test nine suspected foods—one each day. Beginning 30 minutes after each meal, Bob was instructed to give himself a reading and handwriting test.

The first flare-up occurred just after noon on the second day. The nutritionist in charge could not be absolutely certain whether it was caused by the day's breakfast or by the previous night's dinner. For both meals had been eaten within 18 overlapping hours of the flare-up.

A quick look at Bob's reading and writing records confirmed that Bob had experienced blurred vision that had begun about an hour after breakfast that morning and Bob's handwriting had become noticeably shaky and unreadable. On this basis, the nutritionist decided it was the breakfast food that had triggered the arthritis.

Two other flare-ups that followed occurred on rising and were clearly associated with the previous day's food.

Altogether, Bob tested allergy-positive to wheat, rice, and corn. These foods were dropped immediately.

A week later, the pain and swelling in Bob's joints had subsided once more. He strictly followed his dietary instructions and he has been free of arthritis for more than a year.

An Easy Way to Trace Arthritis-Aggravating Food Families

Many people with arthritic disease find they are allergic to several foods, not just one. Some people have shown allergy reactions to as many as 15 or more different foods.

In many cases, people with multiple sensitivities react to several closely related foods that allergists group together in a single family. The food families are related in that all members of one family are recognized by the immune system as having similar "foreign" antigens.

For example, two fairly common arthritis-aggravating allergens, potatoes and tomatoes, both belong to the nightshade family. Many people who are sensitive to tomatoes are also sensitive to potatoes, and vice versa. These people have a predisposed sensitivity towards other members of the nightshade family such as green and red peppers, eggplant, and paprika.

If tests confirm that you are allergic to any food belonging to a common food family, you may well have a cross-sensitivity to other foods in the same family. This knowledge is extremely helpful in tracking down arthritis-aggravating allergens.

For instance, a normal meal might contain both a potato and a tomato. Together, these two are sufficient to induce an arthritic flare-up. But if you omitted either the potato or the tomato, the remaining food may not be sufficient to produce a rejection response by the immune system.

Here are the principal food families. Not all are common allergens. The cruciferous and gourd families are rarely allergenic. And not all members of a food family are allergenic. For instance, the legume peanut is a common allergen, mung beans are not.

Common Food Family Groups

ASTER: artichoke, chamomile, dandelion, endive, escarole, goldenrod, lettuce, safflower oil, sunflower oil, sunflower seeds.

BOVINE: beef, goat, lamb, mutton, veal.

CITRUS: grapefruit, lemon, lime, orange, tangerine, tangelo.

CRUCIFEROUS: broccoli, Brussels sprouts, cabbage, cauliflower, Chinese celery, collards, horseradish, kale, kohlrabi, mustard, mustard greens, radish, rutabagas, turnip.

DAIRY: all milk and dairy products.

GRASS: all cereal grains including bamboo shoots, barley, corn, malt, millet, molasses, oats, rice, rye, sorghum, and wheat. Also sprouts of any of these grains.

GOURD: cantaloupe, cucumber, melons—all types—pumpkin, squash, watermelon, zucchini. Also seeds of these plants.

LEGUMES: alfalfa, mung beans, peanuts, soybean and soy products, all beans and peas, lecithin, and licorice. Also pea, bean, and alfalfa sprouts.

NIGHTSHADE: cayenne pepper, chili pepper, green and red peppers, eggplant, paprika, potato, and tomato.

PARSLEY: anise, carrot, celeriac, celery, chervil, coriander, cumin, dill, fennel, parsnip. Also seeds of these plants.

PLUM: almond, apricot, cherry, nectarine, peach, persimmon, plum, prune, wild cherry.

POULTRY: chicken, goose, and duck meat. Eggs.

ROSE: blackberry, boysenberry, dewberry, loganberry, raspberry, rose hip, strawberry, youngberry.

YEAST: baker's and brewer's yeast.

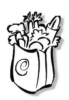

The Worst Arthritis-Aggravating Food

Population studies show that arthritis is most common in countries where wheat is the staple food. Wheat is possibly the most common arthritis aggravating allergen and definitely near the top of the most allergenic food list. Scientists have discovered that many people, including some who have never had arthritis before, experience arthritis symptoms in a relatively short time when an extract of wheat is placed under the tongue.

While it's possible to have a true wheat or grain allergy, it's often the gluten or grain protein that creates symptoms. For some people gluten sensitivity is part of a condition called Celiac Disease where gluten damages part of the intestinal wall. The result is a leaky gut, malabsorption of nutrients, and other digestive problems.

However, not everyone with gluten intolerance has Celiac Disease.

Investigation has shown that it's possible to be sensitive to gluten from other cereal grains. British rheumatology researchers, Drs. Gail Darlington and N. W. Ramsey, say cereals are among the foods most often implicated in producing symptoms in patients with rheumatoid arthritis. Wheat and corn are cited as the worst[39]. (Note that corn is low in gluten. A reaction to corn probably indicates a true corn allergy.) Hence if you show a confirmed sensitivity to wheat or to any other gluten-containing grains, you should suspect all other members of the grass family. Hayfever and allergies to pollens and grasses may create a cross-reactivity including consumed cereals.

Wheat products, which usually provoke the same sensitivity as wheat itself, are found in a wide variety of processed foods such as bread, baked goods, beer, liquor, mayonnaise, pasta, ice cream, and most sausages. (Check the label.) Many alcoholic drinks contain large amounts of various grains as well as sugar and yeast. Corn (free of gluten) and its products are also common ingredients in processed foods.

Notice that the digestive diet plan excludes all gluten-containing grains. Brown rice, millet, amaranth, and quinoa are typical cereals permitted on a gluten-free diet. However, if while eating these foods you're still in pain, consider eliminating them as well and see how you feel.

Other Common Foods That Aggravate Arthritis

The same can be said of soybean and soy products. Processed foods may contain varying amounts of many basic foods, each of which could be allergenic. Which is one reason why you should stay strictly away from *all* processed foods from now on. Soy is a common food additive. (Tofu, tempeh, and other soy-based products are excellent foods if you're not allergic to them.)

The nightshade family is another group of fairly common arthritis-aggravating allergens. Besides provoking an immune response, these foods contain solanine, a glycoalkaloid which inhibits the action of cholinesterase, the enzyme that provides flexibility and agility in muscles.

Although brewer's yeast is recognized as a splendid source of B-complex vitamins, it is also a protein-rich microorganism. Tiny particles of this protein may be recognized as a foreign antigen in the bloodstream. The same is true of baker's yeast used in making most (but not all) breads.

Protein-rich foods like cereal gluten, eggs, yeast, soybeans, and dairy foods are high on the arthritis-promoting allergy list. The safest and most beneficial form of whole protein is a cold-water fish like salmon or haddock.

Starch, lectins, and other food constituents can also induce food allergies. Even preservatives and additives may arouse an allergic response.

Audrey M.'s Food Sleuthing Pays Off by Eliminating Her Arthritis

Audrey M., a 45-year-old nurse, had had rheumatoid arthritis for several years. Through reading medical journals she had become aware of the growing scientific evidence that food allergies are one aggravator of rheumatoid arthritis.

Audrey didn't have time to cleanse but felt certain she was allergic to what she called her "arthritis trigger," a hefty sandwich of lettuce, Swiss cheese, and tomato placed between two slices of whole wheat bread generously spread with peanut butter.

Audrey knew that, except for the fat in the cheese and peanut butter, these were all considered healthful foods. Yet each was also a fairly common arthritis allergen. Moreover one of the sandwiches formed the core of every meal and snack that Audrey ate. Each day, she ate at least six large sandwiches, and often seven or eight.

If a meal or snack didn't include her favorite sandwich, Audrey felt quite uncomfortable. The discomfort would increase until she was able to eat the allergic food once more.

Helping to confirm her suspicions that her digestive tract was beneath all this was the fact that Audrey felt stuffed and gassy soon after eating a sandwich and she experienced frequent diarrhea. After one particularly painful flare-up, Audrey decided to eliminate her arthritis trigger.

Once Audrey actually stopped eating the sandwich, benefits soon began to appear. Within three days, her digestive problems cleared up completely. The pain and swelling in her wrists and knees grew noticeably less.

But a continuous low-level pain lingered on. Audrey knew enough of nutrition to realize it was probably because she was still eating some of the ingredients found in the bread or because she was still eating a food of the same family as those in her sandwich.

Right away, Audrey cut all other foods containing wheat or yeast together with sour cream, potatoes, corn, and soybeans—foods she regularly ate that belonged to the same families as the foods in her sandwich.

A week after dropping all these foods, the last of Audrey's arthritis pain and inflammation disappeared. Later, when she underwent a cleanse and food testing, Audrey found she was sensitive to only half the foods she had eliminated .She discovered she could safely go on eating tomatoes, potatoes, peanuts, and soybeans.

But as a temporary expedient, her makeshift sleuthing proved remarkably successful.

Purging Arthritis or Gout by Eliminating Destructive Foods

By now, you should have identified many of the allergenic foods that are aggravating your arthritic disease. Or if any doubt exists as to which of two overlapping foods are allergenic, you can test each one again by the alternative tests described in Chapter 9. Likewise, if you were unable to test all the foods on your list, you can test the remainder the same way.

In any case, by eliminating *all* of these foods from your diet—including those you have not yet tested or confirmed—and repairing your GI tract, you should be well on the way towards ending the pain, stiffness, and inflammation arising from rheumatoid and similar forms of arthritic disease caused by poor digestion that often underlies food intolerances. As osteoarthritis and gout pain may also be worsened by an ailing intestine, eliminating the responsible allergenic foods may significantly help to reduce pain from these diseases.

To completely overcome gout, you must cut out all stressor foods together with the special gout-aggravating foods listed in Chapter 11, and you must bring your weight back down to normal.

To completely overcome osteoarthritis, you must cut out all the stressor foods described in Chapter 11 and bring your weight down to normal.

 ## How Other Food Testing Methods Can Help

What if you completely overlooked an allergenic food while compiling your list of suspected foods? The food would not have been tested and you might still be eating it every day. As a result, arthritis pain would still be with you.

If you have any type of arthritis other than gout or osteoarthritis and if pain, stiffness, and inflammation have continued after the cleanse and through the food-testing period, this may be the explanation.

You can easily test any suspect foods you may have overlooked by using the alternative techniques described in the next chapter.

Meanwhile, once your tests are over and you have eliminated both stressor and allergenic foods from your diet, you can go ahead and combine any number of compatible foods to form any meal that you desire.

If you want to pursue other natural arthritis treatments, ask for help from a practitioner trained in this area. (See Appendix C.)

Chapter *9*

Picking the Best Food Allergy Test for You— Including More Self-Help Methods

---

Elizabeth D. was one of hundreds of arthritis sufferers interviewed for this book who had retired to the Southwest in the hope of finding relief from the dry climate. Elizabeth did eventually find relief, though not through low humidity.

"I first had pain and swelling in my hands, then it spread to my elbows, shoulders, and knees," she told me. "My doctor diagnosed it as rheumatoid arthritis. He placed me on 15 aspirin a day. That didn't help, so he gave me Indocin™ and later a steroid. They helped briefly but only in large doses.

"At 47 I could barely walk a block without crippling pain. I'd lost 25 pounds and I was as thin as a rake. So my husband retired here after 30 years in the service. We thought the climate might help. But that was another disappointment.

"Then I got pneumonia. Our new family physician here said it was because the steroid I was taking suppressed my immune system so much that I had no resistance. I also found that the steroid was causing bone loss. And the 15 daily aspirin were causing severe gastritis and ringing in my ears.

"The drugs had me really scared! Not far away is an arthritis clinic. They use fasting to find out which foods cause arthritis. I didn't really believe in it at all. But I was so desperate I got my husband to drive me there. They said I was too thin to fast, but they did have an alternative method.

"They used a pulse test that somebody developed back in the 1930s. Whenever you eat a food that you're sensitive to, your pulse rate rises. Of course, you have to stop taking medication. The whole thing was so simple I could have done it myself at home. Anyway, they found I was allergic to beef, eggs, milk, chocolate, pork, and luncheon meats.

"Of course, they didn't know which of these was actually causing arthritis. So they told me to cut all of them out of my diet. They also gave me a list of high-risk foods to avoid and another list of natural foods I should eat instead.

"Well, I never really believed it would work, but I followed their advice anyway. Believe it or not, after a month on this food, the pain and swelling in my joints started to die down. After three months, I could walk a mile without pain. My weight gradually came back up to normal.

"The only flare-up I've had was when we went to a dude ranch for a week and I went on a beef kick. I swear I'll never do anything like it again. It undid the work of months. This time, I'm sticking right to my diet. Besides, it helps me stay completely regular, I'm 52 now. I'm completely free of arthritis and I feel twice as good as I ever did before."

All Allergy Foods Should Be Eliminated

Elizabeth's recovery is typical of many of the people in this book where, for one reason or another, a fast or cleanse could not be used. If you are unable or unwilling to cleanse or to fast, or if you cannot spare the time, there *are* alternatives. The self-help food tests don't necessarily tell you exactly which foods are aggravating arthritis, but they are a starting point. For more precise results, see the roster of lab tests at the end of this chapter.

Whether or not a food sensitivity is causing arthritis, it's wise to cut it out anyway.

Before we go on, we'd like to emphasize this. Don't be tempted to bypass the cleansing diet and use one or another of the alternative self-help tests because they sound easier. They are second choice alternatives, not substitutes.

None will improve intestinal health or reduce rheumatoid arthritis pain like a cleansing regimen and healthy dietary changes. Nor do they magnify test reactions to reveal low level food allergies that may be aggravating arthritis.

How Your Pulse Can Reveal Hidden Food Allergies

One alternative test for food sensitivity is the pulse test. This method was first developed in the 1930s by Dr. Arthur Coca, a famous immunologist. When his wife became ill, Dr. Coca discovered that she became worse after eating specific foods which increased her pulse rate. When these foods were eliminated, his wife recovered.

Other allergists have refined and improved the method since. But the technique is still basically the one developed by Dr. Coca. While this test has its drawbacks—not all pulse increases are due to food allergies and not all allergies increase your pulse—you can do it yourself at home with fair results.

Before you can use the pulse test, you must first establish your normal pulse rate and your normal pulse limits. To do so, take your pulse 14 times a day for three consecutive days immediately prior to testing the foods.

As a preliminary, practice feeling your pulse a few times with the tips of your middle and index fingers. Your pulse is located on the underside of your forearm about an inch above the wrist on the thumb side. Practice taking your pulse several times for 30 seconds while you time yourself with the second hand of a watch or clock or with a digital timepiece that shows seconds. If you count 35 beats in 30 seconds, your pulse rate is 70 beats per minute ($2 \times 35 = 70$).

Finding Your Normal Pulse Rate

To establish your normal pulse rate you must read your pulse for three consecutive days immediately prior to food testing like this:

1. Immediately on waking and while still lying in bed.

2. Immediately prior to each meal.

3. At 30, 60, and 90 minutes after each meal.

4. Immediately before retiring.

Except when taking your pulse in bed as you awaken, take all the other readings while seated. Note down the time and number of beats for each reading in a notebook.

Here is an example:

	Day 1	Day 2	Day 3
On rising	60	59	59
Before breakfast	58	57	60
30 minutes after breakfast	68	67	68
60 minutes after breakfast	74	70	74
90 minutes after breakfast	70	66	70
Before lunch	63	62	66
30 minutes after lunch	74	71	74
60 minutes after lunch	76	72	77
90 minutes after lunch	70	67	75
Before dinner	68	62	65
30 minutes after dinner	77	68	76
60 minutes after dinner	75	70	79
90 minutes after dinner	73	67	77
On retiring	70	63	70
Daily totals	976	921	990
	÷14	÷14	÷14
Average daily rate	69.7	65.7	70.7
Normal pulse rate	69		
Daily high	77	72	79
Daily low	58	57	59

Differential	19	15	20
Normal high rate	76		

To find your daily average rate, total the 14 daily readings and divide by 14.

To find your normal daily pulse rate, total the average daily pulse rates for each of the three days and divide by three. (Example: 69.7 + 65.7 + 70.7 = 206.1 ÷ 3 = 68.7 which we round off to 69.)

To find your daily differential, subtract the lowest reading of each day from the highest reading of each day. (Example for Day 1: 77 - 58 = 19.)

To find your normal high rate, total the three daily high rates and divide by three (Example: 77 + 72 + 79 = 228 ÷ 3 = 76).

Your Pulse Indicates Your Inner Health

Now examine the pulse readings in your notebook for each of the three days.

If on any day, the difference between the highest and lowest readings exceeds 16, it may indicate sensitivity to a food that you ate that day. If this difference on any day is below 16, no food sensitivity is indicated.

If the average daily high reading varies from day to day by more than two, it again indicates a possible food sensitivity. If the daily high rate remains constant, it probably means you are not sensitive to any foods you ate during the three-day period.

In our sample pulse observations, two readings indicate the probability of one or more food sensitivities. For example, on two days, a difference of more than 16 indicates a possibility that at least one allergenic food was eaten on two out of three days.

Again, the variation in the daily high rate exceeds 16, again indicating the possible existence of a food sensitivity.

If your notes show that your pulse rose to more than six beats per minute over and above your normal pulse rate after eating any particular food, test those foods first.

In your notebook you must also record the basic food contents of all foods you eat at each meal, including any beverages. Snacks, beverages, or chewing gum should not be taken between meals as they may distort pulse readings.

Preparing for the Pulse Test

Take your pulse only after you have been seated for several minutes. If you find a high reading, be sure it is not due to exercise, emotional stress, excitement, infection or infectious disease, or severe sunburn. Any sudden increase *not* due to one of these causes may be due to a sensitivity to a food or to an environmental allergy.

You can usually detect a sensitivity due to something in the environment such as dust, pollen, animal danders, or chemicals because your pulse will remain high the entire time you remain in that environment. If this happens, try changing your environment while you continue to eat the same foods. If you had an environmental allergy, your pulse rate should gradually drop back to normal. If your pulse rate remains high, it could mean you are allergic to one or more of the foods you are eating.

All prerequisites that applied to food testing after a cleanse apply equally to pulse testing. You must first make a list of suspect foods to be tested (Chapter 7) and you should avoid testing stressor foods. Only basic foods should be tested.

All smoking and non-essential medication should be stopped at least three days prior to establishing your normal pulse rate and they must be withheld throughout the food tests that follow. Any food to be tested must have been eaten regularly and at least once during the five days preceding the pulse tests.

If while establishing your normal pulse rate, your notes show that your pulse rose to more than 10 beats over and above your normal pulse rate after eating any particular foods, test those foods first.

All foods to be tested should be prepared as described in Chapter 7 for the challenge test. Unlike the cleansing program, you eat and test only one food at a time. But with the pulse test you can test as many as two foods in one day—one at a time, of course—each at breakfast and lunch.

Mini-Meals Give Best Results

Prepare a normal sized meal of the single food to be tested. Divide that meal into three equal portions. And eat each portion 60 minutes apart.

There's one important rule to observe: if immediately prior to the time when you should eat the next mini-meal, your pulse is reading above its normal daily rate, postpone eating until it drops to normal or below and has stayed in that range for a full hour.

Suppose you were testing wheat and beef. Assuming it takes 10 minutes to eat a mini-meal, your eating schedule might look like this:

7:30 A.M.	Wheat
8:40 A.M.	Wheat
9:50 A.M.	Wheat
12:30 P.M.	Beef
1:40 P.M.	Beef
2:50 P.M.	Beef
6:30 P.M.	Normal dinner without suspected food allergies or stressor foods

You would eat at these times only if your pulse reads normal or below. The advantage of eating small mini-meals is that the amount of food is not sufficiently large to cause any significant increase in heart rate due to the added task of digestion. At all times, only pure water should be drunk. Any suspected beverage must be tested as though it were a food as described in Chapter 7.

If your pulse is above normal at any time you are scheduled to begin another mini-meal, wait for it to drop to normal. Then allow it to beat for one full hour at the normal rate or lower before you eat. If your pulse remains high or allergy-related symptoms persist into the evening, postpone pulse testing for a day.

Now for the actual food testing.

What Your Pulse Tells About the Foods You Eat

Go ahead and eat your first mini-meal.

Immediately after eating, take your pulse and record it, together with a notation of the time and the food you are testing, in your notebook. Also note any unusual symptoms over the next half hour.

Do the same thing 30 minutes later.

Now, compare your pulse rate immediately after eating with the rate 30 minutes later.

If it has increased by 16 beats per minute or more, this indicates a strong possibility that you are sensitive to the test food.

If at the 30-minute reading your pulse reads 10 beats or more per minute above your normal high rate, this again indicates a possibility of sensitivity to the test food.

If both events occur together, you can regard this as a possible indication of a strong sensitivity.

Again, if 30 minutes after the test meal your pulse reads 84 beats per minute or higher, this is another possible indication that you have eaten an allergenic food.

When interpreting these results, be sure of course that you are free of any emotional stress, excitement, infection, heavy sunburn, or the effects of recent exercise. Another confounding factor is delayed reactions to foods. The pulse test works best for more immediate responses to food.

Repeat this process with each mini-meal of the day.

For each test food, compare results for each of the three mini-meals. If any sensitivity indications were repeated two or three times, this is probable proof that your immune system has a strong response to that food.

That food should be dropped from your diet, at least until you have a chance to confirm the sensitivity by another method.

Provided you have eaten the test food regularly right up to the date your food testing begins, you can continue testing suspect foods for five more full days. Just to make this clear, you can continue to eat suspect foods freely during the three days you are establishing your normal pulse rate. The five days we're talking about begin with your first day of actual food testing.

On this basis and assuming no delays, you should be able to test 10 different foods during the five test days.

A Simple Diet Change Brings Speedy Relief to Doreen P.'s Pain-Crippled Knee

Can self-help tests actually help get rid of arthritis?

"The pain was like a sword driven through my knee," this is a 54-year-old woman speaking.

"It was so bad I could not place any weight on my left knee at all. I had to give up driving and stay at home."

Can you imagine such excruciating agony? But that was three years ago. The lady now is a picture of glowing good health. Standing beside the swimming pool at a large Arizona adult community, Doreen P. had just swum a mile non-stop.

"But three years ago, I was crippled by rheumatoid arthritis. My physician started me off with 14 aspirins a day. Then he tried cortisone. But the side effects were so disturbing I had to go back to aspirin.

"We'd heard about cleansing, fasting, and elimination diets. But the arthritis left me completely emaciated. Fasting was out of the question.

"Then a friend told us about a naturopathic doctor who was getting good results with arthritis without fasting. My husband drove me to see him. In one long afternoon session he taught us the basics of sound nutrition. Then he taught us how to use the pulse test and the kinesiology method for testing food.

"We did the tests ourselves at home. The pulse test showed that I was allergy-positive to sugar, milk, beef, chicken, chocolate, and coffee—favorite foods that I'd eaten all my life. The kinesiology tests confirmed the results.

"I hated to give up those foods I loved. But four weeks later I was walking without pain. You couldn't have got me to eat any of those foods again for a million dollars.

"Eventually, by trial and error we found that only the sugar, milk, chocolate, and coffee were causing arthritis. The beef and chicken didn't seem to be causing anything in particular. So I just eat them occasionally, once in a while.

"Right after that my husband retired. We moved here and I haven't had a touch of arthritis since."

A Quick Method for Testing Any Food

At any time when you have met the requirements for food testing, you can use this quick pulse test to check out any food in under an hour. You can do so without having to establish your normal pulse rate in advance.

The requirements are that you must have eaten the test food at least once within the previous five days. You must not have smoked or taken any drugs within three days or any stimulant such as alcohol or coffee for at least 24 hours. You must feel free of emotional stress, excitement, infection, heavy sunburn, or the effects of exercise. And you must be free of the effects of any environmental allergy.

You will get a stronger reaction if you last ate the test food exactly five days previously and have not eaten it since.

The test must be made on an empty stomach. Hence it is best made at breakfast time.

Begin by taking your pulse a few minutes after rising. Take it while seated.

Then eat a light meal of the test food. The amount to eat is about half the size of a regular breakfast. Eat nothing but the test food and drink nothing but pure water.

After eating, wait 30 minutes and take your pulse. If after eating your pulse has risen by 15–20 beats per minute over the reading you got before the meal, this is a fair indication of a sensitivity to that food.

Provided the requirements are always met, you can repeat this test once at breakfast time on any day. The test can help serve to confirm previous tests.

The Quick Pulse Test Helps John L. Identify the Cause of His Arthritis

The quick pulse test is essentially the same technique that helped John L. locate the cause of his arthritis.

"I'd *been* to an arthritis clinic. I'd *learned* all about fasting, nutrition, and natural foods. I'd *changed* my diet completely. But I *still* had rheumatoid arthritis."

John L., a former Navy officer who was forced to retire because of arthritis, tells this story.

"They'd told me at the clinic that I shouldn't smoke or drink beer. Of course, everyone knows that smoking is bad for health. But I just couldn't see how smoking or alcohol could affect arthritis."

John described how he found a book on pulse testing for food allergies written years ago.

"All you had to do was to eat a meal of just one food and take your pulse 30 minutes later. Well, one day I noticed that after a cigarette my pulse rate rose 18 beats a minute. After two cans of beer it rose 22 beats a minute. According to the book, these were danger signals.

"It scared the daylights out of me! I quit smoking and drinking right there, cold turkey! Three weeks later, my arthritis faded away.

"I did have three flare-ups afterwards. But the last was five years ago. I've stuck with the diet and I've steered clear of cigarettes and beer and I've been totally free of arthritis ever since."

How to Tap into Your Body's Instinctual Wisdom

There's an even swifter method for testing for food sensitivity. This simple test, called applied kinesiology (AK), works on the principle that the body knows what may be wrong with it and what needs to be done to restore health. A branch of conventional medicine that studies muscle motion is also called kinesiology. This is different from AK or applied kinesiology discussed here.

AK isn't so far-fetched. When animals get sick, they listen to their instinctual body wisdom which tells them to stop eating and to fast. Cleansing frees the body from the task of digestion and permits self-healing to proceed at the fastest possible rate.

Studies have also shown that if given the choice of a wide variety of basic foods (no sugar, sweets, ice cream, or other junk food) both animals and children will automatically select those foods containing the nutritional elements that their body needs most.

To use kinesiology, we must learn to read the signals our body gives us. When we feed our body a food which the immune system rejects, say AK practitioners, the body will let us know right away that this sensitivity exists.

AK's appeal lies in its fast, cheap, and relatively easy application. This science, developed by Detroit chiropractor George Goodheart in 1964, is relatively new. Many practitioners, including those of the natural medical persuasion, say AK is too subjective to be of use. Others say more research needs to be done. Applied kinesiologists say their science is more complex to learn than people originally thought, and only a trained professional will obtain accurate results[40].

However, our purpose in writing this book is to give you beginning tips on how to improve your arthritis, including assessing food allergies. By all means, give kinesiology a try—many have used it successfully. Just remember, the answers you get are limited.

How to Put Test Foods into Your Bloodstream in Seconds

Kinesiology theory says we can learn how well the body tolerates any particular food by observing a reflex that exists between the tongue, immune system, and brain. The effect of this reflex is said to reduce muscle strength throughout the body. Applied kinesiology is also called muscle testing.

This phenomenon has been compared to nitroglycerine, a medicine used every day by tens of millions of heart disease patients all over the U.S .and throughout the world to relieve angina attacks.

An angina attack is an unbearable pain in the chest that foreshadows a heart attack. People with heart disease suffer frequently from these pains. Any angina attack can develop into a heart attack. To prevent a heart attack, doctors prescribe nitroglycerine tablets to be taken at the first sign of angina pain. The nitroglycerine relaxes blood vessels and prevents the blockage of a coronary artery that would otherwise precipitate a heart attack.

When an angina pain occurs, a heart attack may follow in just two or three minutes. Somehow, that nitroglycerine has to be placed in the bloodstream in mere seconds. The pain of angina is such that a victim could not possibly inject the nitroglycerine himself. And if simply swallowed, it would take 10–15 minutes to enter the bloodstream.

Instead, at the first hint of angina pain, a nitroglycerine tablet is placed *under the tongue.* Here it is immediately absorbed into the bloodstream, and within seconds it reaches the coronary arteries.

Kinesiologists say not only nitroglycerine but *any* food placed under the tongue is absorbed into the body immediately. It is through this same access that tiny particles of undigested food enter the bloodstream and provoke a rejectivity response. Other more numerous particles are absorbed later through the intestines.

A Simple Kinesiology Technique That Helps Identify Aggravating Foods

When the immune system rejects particles of a non-tolerated food, a neurological reflex relays this information to the brain. The brain, explain AK theorists, reacts by reducing the strength and power in our body muscles. The entire process works about as swiftly, and in somewhat the same way as the knee jerk reflex.

Within 30 seconds of placing a sample of test food under the tongue, we supposedly lose an appreciable degree of muscular strength.

This is how kinesiology food testing is said to work. By placing a sample of the test food under the tongue, a person's sensitivity to that food can be detected by simply measuring muscle strength 30–90 seconds later.

The same requirements are necessary for kinesiological testing as for pulse or cleansing tests. No smoking or drugs during the preceding three days and no coffee or alcohol within 24 hours. Any food to be tested should have been eaten fairly regularly and at least once during the preceding five days. And you should be emotionally calm, relaxed, and feeling well.

The tests should be made on a relatively empty stomach. Thus we suggest doing any kinesiological testing before eating the first meal of the day.

Reading Your Body's Danger Signals

To conduct a test, you need a second person.

Begin by holding out your arm horizontally to the side, palm down. Keep the arm firm, straight, and rigid.

The other person then grasps your wrist with one hand and gently rests his other hand on your shoulder. He then presses firmly and steadily downward with his first hand until your arm is forced down to your side. It must be done smoothly and without jerking. The tester gauges the strength required to overcome your resistance.

Next, lower your arm and chew a small piece of test food. Masticate it and mix it well with saliva. Then place it under your tongue and keep it there until the test is over. Let exactly 60 seconds tick away on your watch.

Then hold your arm out again and have the tester press it down to your side. If your resistance weakens appreciably, this is marked as a food sensitivity. If your muscle strength remains constant, the food is not counted as an allergen.

Immediately when the test is over, rinse the food out of your mouth. Don't swallow it.

If you got no reaction you can continue testing with another food. If the food tested allergy positive, sit down and rest for 10 minutes before testing the next food.

At any one session you can test half a dozen different foods. More than that, and your muscles become tired merely from holding your arm up in the air. This increases the chance of flawed results.

To test a liquid, take a mouthful, work it around your mouth for 15 seconds until well mixed with saliva, then hold it under the tongue as if it were food. Any beverages should be prepared double strength.

As with all other food testing methods, keep detailed notes of all test results together with dates and times. If you detect any sensitivities, you can recheck them again later or the following day for confirmation.

Claudia A. Lets Her Body's Own Wisdom Guide Her to Freedom from Arthritis

Many years ago Claudia A. hit her right knee on a desk. Arthritis pains soon began. Within months, pain and inflammation spread to the fingers and wrist of her right hand. Her doctor prescribed large doses of aspirin, but her joints still felt as though they were on fire, and every morning her hand and leg were painfully stiff.

Claudia jumped at the chance to try kinesiology and food elimination. She made a list of foods she craved most. To let the stiffness work out of her joints, she did the testing in mid-afternoon. Claudia skipped breakfast and lunch and took the test on an empty stomach.

Claudia didn't have much muscle strength left. But a distinct weakening occurred after she took mouthfuls of sugar, wheat, egg, and cheese.

She was advised to try cutting out these foods along with several other health robbing stressor foods. And, of course, to stay off aspirin.

A month later, a cheerful Claudia reported her arthritis was much improved. She could move her knee and hand without pain, but there were heavy cracking noises. She continued eating natural foods and practiced gentle exercises to improve joint mobility.

Three months later she could use her formerly crippled hand and was walking again and doing housework and had totally recovered.

Confirming Allergies with Alternative Tests

Any of the tests described in this chapter may be used to confirm the results of other tests. For example, if the elimination-challenge test shows a sensitivity to beef, wheat, and chocolate, you can confirm these results with the pulse and kinesiology tests.

Since neither the pulse nor kinesiology tests are as sensitive as the elimination-challenge test, we suggest using both methods to test your list of suspect foods.

If you have any doubts about foods you may eat in the future, you can give them a quick preliminary check out with the quick pulse test or the kinesiology method.

For greater certainty, you can also test any suspect food at second or third time, using the quick pulse test or the kinesiology method.

Off to the Doctor's Office for Allergy Tests

We've already offered many do-it-yourself food allergy tests. But if you're unable or unwilling to carry them out, or would rather be under the supervision of a professional experienced in testing and treating food allergies, that's fine too. After speaking with several natural health practitioners, we found that opinions vary on what's the best test. Here are brief descriptions of the most popular laboratory and office tests, and how accurate they are.

Skin Test

If you've ever had respiratory allergies to pollen or animal fur, you probably know about the skin test. This conventional allergy test uses your forearm or back as a pin cushion where small amounts of suspected allergic substances are pricked or scratched into your skin.

This is a wonderful way to test fixed or immediate allergic reactions, including to some foods. According to Dr. Thomas Golbert, from the University of Colorado School of Medicine in Denver and contributing author to *Allergic Diseases: Diagnosis and Management* (41), most food allergies are the immediate type. In his opinion, delayed food allergies are infrequent and systemic reactions (like arthritis) to food allergies are "rare."

Many (if not most) natural health practitioners would disagree with Dr. Golbert's judgment that most food allergies are fixed. And for that reason, the rather uncomfortable skin test is ill-suited for detecting hidden food allergies.

The ELISA Laboratory Test

ELISA isn't the name of a girl. It stands for enzyme-linked immunosorbent assay, a type of food allergy test. Blood is drawn and tested for antibodies against certain foods. Both fixed and delayed food allergies can be tested this way. Like any blood test, the ELISA isn't perfect and may be too costly for some (check with your health insurance company about reimbursement). But it will pick up several food allergies without the fuss and muss of the elimination-challenge test and is more accurate than the pulse test and kinesiology.

The Cytotoxic Test

The cytotoxic test is based on the idea that when food extracts are added to a blood sample, the allergens will damage white blood cells. This damage is viewed through a microscope by a lab technician and recorded over a two hour period. This blood test, popular several years ago, has fallen somewhat out of favor. Although cheaper than the ELISA and related allergy tests, its results are too subjective to be of use.

ElectroAcupuncture According to Voll

Interest in this method of food allergy testing, also called EAV, has climbed during the last few years possibly due to its noninvasive manner. While the patient holds a negatively charged electrode in one hand (it won't shock you), the EAV operator places a positive electrode on various acupuncture points over the patient's body. A tray of bottles that hold food extracts are rigged into the EAV circuitry for testing. Readings on the EAV machine indicate the presence of food allergies or sensitivities.

This is still a controversial method of food allergy testing, even within the natural health field. More research is needed.

The Provocation-Neutralization and Serial-Dilution Test

The PN-SD test is a favorite of clinical ecologists, doctors who specialize in treating environmental illness. Like the skin test, food allergies are diagnosed by scratching the skin with allergenic extracts. Symptoms are then watched for. PN-SD proponents claim that certain dilutions of an allergic substance evokes reactions, while other dilutions alleviate or neutralize symptoms. When that perfect alleviating diluted dose is found, it's used as a treatment. (Something like allergy shots.)

Another version of this test involves placing allergenic extracts under the tongue, appropriate for children. Many doctors are skeptical of this subjective and time consuming test. More concrete research is required before it's fully accepted.

Stressor Foods That Pave the Way for Arthritic Disease

The first step in recovering from any form of arthritic disease is to stop eating all stressor foods. Stressor foods are those problem foods that tear down your health and pave the way for arthritis.

We call them stressor foods because they are so harmful to health that eating them places a stress on the body. When we continue to eat stressor foods over a period of years, the continued stress throws the body out of balance and we become sickly and run down.

While arthritis is often genetically predetermined, healthy people don't get arthritis as frequently because healthy people don't eat stressor foods.

Arthritic disease usually occurs after years of harmful eating habits have led to physical harm to the joints and lowered the body's resistance.

How Good Is Your Health, Really?

While natural health practitioners use diagnostic tests on their patients, they understand good health goes far beyond merely checking OK on a battery of laboratory read-outs and being free of any discernible sign of disease.

"I always relied on my doctor to tell me how healthy I was," this was a 52-year-old woman speaking. "He told me I was in good health. But a month later I was stricken by arthritis."

When we questioned Emily J., we learned that despite her doctor's reassurance, she was far from being in optimum health when arthritis first appeared. Her diet consisted almost entirely of canned and convenience foods, white bread, fried dishes, and sugar-filled desserts.

As a result of the stress these foods had placed on her body, Emily J. was 25 pounds overweight, had frequent gastrointestinal distress, was unable to walk for more than 10 minutes, and suffered from frequent colds and infections. Yet because she showed no symptoms of major disease, her doctor gave Emily J. a clean bill of health.

Like virtually everyone who is stricken with arthritis, Emily J. was eating poorly. She had chronic constipation and frequent indigestion. By natural standards she was in mediocre health. But a medical check up had failed to find anything wrong.

Arthritis does not usually attack people in optimum health. It frequently takes years of eating stressor foods that upset body chemistry by raising cholesterol and blood fat levels, creating poor digestion and elimination, causing overweight and skeletal bone loss, and by weakening joints and their ability to regenerate.

 Foods That Kill

Stressor foods are the same killer foods that contribute to other degenerative diseases including heart disease, hypertension, diabetes, and even some forms of cancer. No one can continue to eat stressor foods and remain permanently healthy.

The first step in recovery from arthritis is to drop all stressor foods from the diet *now and for always!*

Stressor Foods Prevent Jerry B.'s Body from Healing Itself

Jerry B. didn't believe it was necessary to cut out stressor foods to recover from arthritis. Jerry had rheumatoid arthritis for five years. He underwent food testing at an arthritis clinic and tested allergy-positive to wheat, beef, milk, potatoes, tomatoes, and caffeine. Jerry stopped eating these allergenic foods and a few weeks later his arthritis began to disappear.

Although Jerry was told at the clinic to stop eating all stressor foods, he believed this wasn't really necessary.

"Why?" he asked himself. "I've stopped eating the foods I'm allergic to. My arthritis is gone."

But Jerry did not remain arthritis-free for long. Although some of the allergenic foods he had cut out were also stressor foods, he went right on eating other stressor foods. Nor did Jerry begin to eat the health building restorative foods that would have made him well.

The result was that Jerry's nutritional stress remained uncorrected. His poor digestion and leaky gut created an intolerance for other common foods that remained in his diet.

A few months after his arthritis cleared up, it was right back again.

As in Jerry's case, even though we stop eating all allergy-causing foods, we remain nutritionally depleted if we continue to eat stressor foods. We may even build new sensitivities to other common foods because the intestinal tract isn't doing its job.

Our Chemicalized, Mass-Produced Imitation Food

A basic arthritis aggravator are the stressor foods in our typical American diet. The foods that most of us are eating at every meal are slowly killing us.

Actually, it is not so much the food itself that makes us sick but the way it is raised and prepared. Our ancestors did not get heart disease because their meat came from wild game or from lean, unfattened steers bred on the range. Today, we eat marbled steaks from steers force-fed in fattening pens where they are routinely given hormones to make them fatter still.

Raw cow's milk seldom tests out allergy-positive. But modern homogenized milk contains an enzyme called xanthine oxidase that scars artery walls and heart tissue, causing cholesterol deposits and giving rise to hardening of the arteries, hypertension, strokes, and heart attack. Homogenization also destroys the desirable enzyme phosphatase plus essential B-vitamins and vitamin C.

The wheat our ancestors ate was a perfectly wholesome food. But around 1900, millers discovered that refined flour would keep longer than whole wheat flour and bring in more profit. Refining removes the germ of wheat, including all its fiber, and leaches out almost all vitamins and minerals. Prior to 1900, heart disease, appendicitis, and hiatal hernias were rare. Today, diverticulosis—an ailment caused by refined foods and lack of fiber—is a common disease among adult Americans while one of every two Americans over 50 suffers from varicose veins or hemorrhoids—other diseases caused by foods low in fiber.

These same degenerative diseases, including arthritis, appear in every country that adopts the western industrialized diet that most people eat in America. The plain fact is that 60 percent of calories most of us eat consists of just two foods: fat and sugar.

The western diet with its deadly amounts of fat and sugar, its distressing lack of fiber, and its proclivity for processes rather than whole foods has spread to every industrialized country. Until recently, the Japanese lived on a far more natural diet and their incidence of degenerative diseases, including arthritis, was far below ours. But the Japanese are rapidly adopting the western diet and, as they do, their rate of arthritis, gout, heart disease, diabetes, and cancer has soared.

Counterfeit Foods—Our Disastrous Diet

Government statistics reveal the changing food picture in the U.S. In 1938, the average American ate 120 pounds of meat a year. Now we eat 160 pounds. Today, we eat 27 percent fewer fresh vegetables and 39 percent fewer fresh fruits than in 1938.

Not to be totally pessimistic, the nutrition lessons of the last two decades haven't fallen on deaf ears. Americans are opting for more fish and chicken over red meat. And with the rising popularity of Mexican and East Indian foods, beans, particularly pinto and navy, are consumed at an increasing rate.

Still, in the modern diet, more than half the food is processed, while such basic foods as meat and poultry are dangerously tampered with long before they reach the processing stage.

Research shows that almost everyone who suffers from arthritis is a heavy eater of refined carbohydrates (white flour and sugar) and foods dangerously high in saturated fats such as whole-fat dairy products, steak, eggs, and other fatty forms of animal protein. Many arthritis patients are also steady consumers of fast, convenience foods.

The same research also shows that native Africans, who eat no refined foods at all and who still live entirely on fresh, whole natural foods, seldom suffer from arthritis or from any other degenerative disease.

The same is true among vegetarians in the U.S. Vegans, those who not only abstain from rich meats but also from eggs and dairy foods, scarcely experience any form of arthritic disease. Nor do they often get heart disease, diabetes, cancer, osteoporosis, diverticulosis, varicose veins, appendicitis, hiatal hernias, and the long melancholy litany of other degenerative diseases all aggravated by stressor foods.

Or it may be that anyone who chooses to eat vegetarian meals is merely health conscious. It may be that the beneficial anti-inflammatory omega-3 fats and extra fiber found in wholesome, intact foods is key, not necessarily avoiding meat at all costs.

At any rate, as the Africans and vegetarians prove, when we feed our bodies the kind of natural foods on which man thrived over millions of years, we remain healthy and free of most degenerative diseases. But overloading our digestive tract with saturated fats, excessive animal protein, and refined foods is like feeding gasoline to a wood stove.

Our bodies are simply not adapted to the foods we eat today, many of which are altered with irradiation or poisoned with chemicals. When we insist on punishing our bodies with stressor foods, it's like buying a one-way ticket to self-destruction.

The U.S. Government Recognizes the Risks of Stressor Foods

The U.S. Government even recommends a drastic reduction in the stressor foods in our diet. When the Surgeon General and U.S. Department of Health and Human Services issued their first ever *Report on Nutrition and Health* a few years ago, its recommendations involved a significant reduction in fats and refined foods.

The *Alternative Diet Book* published by the National Institute of Health recommends major reductions in meat, egg yolks, lard, organ meats, buttermilk, poultry skin, dairy products, and all forms of saturated (mainly animal) fats.

This and the more recent Food Guide Pyramid (replacing the archaic Five Basic Food Groups) recommend that grains, vegetables, and fruits form your dietary foundation. The Pyramid adds dry beans and nuts to its normal protein category of meat, poultry, and fish, and shoves fats and sweets to the "use sparingly" section. The National Institutes of Health diet plan suggests cutting down the excessive amounts of animal protein with which most of us overload our systems. Fish and poultry, it says, are safer foods than red meat.

Past Surgeon General, C. Everett Koop, M.D., states: "Food is necessary for good health." His report found poor diet plays a starring role in half of the 10 leading causes of death for Americans (namely heart disease, cancer, stroke, diabetes, and atherosclerosis). Alcohol contributes to at least three others: suicide, accidents, and chronic liver disease[42].

Literally hundreds of similar studies carried out in every country from Finland to England, Israel, and Japan say the same thing.

At Oldways Preservation & Exchange Trust in Cambridge, Massachusetts, nutritional wisdom from many cultures is preserved and rearranged into modern day dietary guidelines. Working with such prestigious institutions as the Harvard School of Public Health and Cornell University, Oldways has developed both the Mediterranean and Asian Diet Pyramid charts. These nutritional blueprints are laid out much the same way as the Food Guide Pyramid except they take into account healthy Asian and Mediterranean eating styles.

The most striking difference between the American pyramid and these others is that the Asian and Mediterranean cultures treat red meat as a condiment, to be only eaten a couple of times each *month*. Fish, poultry, dairy, and eggs are relegated to the several times a *week* category[43].

For many degenerative diseases begin in the same way: through nutritional stress that distorts normal bodily operations and structure. When saturated fats clog blood vessels, we get heart disease and hypertension. When the pancreas is exhausted from poor nutrient choices, we may get diabetes. When poor diet suppresses the immune system, we are prone to cancer. A dysfunction in the digestive system points to diverticulosis. When an abnormality appears in calcium metabolism, bone loss accelerates and osteoporosis may result.

Among all degenerative diseases is arthritis the *only* exception? The facts show that it is not.

When the immune system is challenged by nutrient-bare foods and other stresses, rheumatoid and similar forms of arthritis together with a variety of related autoimmune diseases are more likely in genetically primed people. When we eat fat-laden stressor foods and become overweight, we're more apt to get osteoarthritis. When we become overweight and eat rich foods high in purines, gout is plausible.

The evidence is clear and unmistakable. The message of almost all modern nutritional research is to cut down on stresssor foods, saturated fats, refined foods, and excessive animal protein to keep joints healthy.

 Alice W. Recovers from Double Arthritis When She Eliminates All Stressor Foods

How successful this step can be was demonstrated by Alice W., a Florida mobile home park resident. Lean, suntanned, and athletic, at 58 Alice looked a glowing picture of robust health. But 10

years earlier, she had been diagnosed as having both osteo and rheumatoid arthritis.

"I was so weak, I could scarcely open a door," she reported. "Each morning, my hands and fingers were so stiff I had to soak them in hot water before I could dress. I was in constant pain and my doctor had prescribed the maximum dosage of steroids.

"I was 40 pounds overweight, but the doctor never mentioned diet. I went right on drinking six colas each day and stuffing myself full of hamburgers, hot dogs, white bread, ice cream, and cheese.

"The doctor told me I would never recover, so I began reading nutritional magazines. I soon discovered there *were* alternatives to drugs. I also learned I'd have to act fast if I were ever to get better. So I took the plunge and enrolled at a natural hygiene institution."

Alice paused to explain that natural hygiene—meaning the Science of natural health—is one of the original natural health care systems.

"The hygienists use fasting for purification but do not test foods for allergies," she said. "They started me out with a five-day water fast, then put me on a diet that drastically reduced fat and cut out just about all fats, refined foods, and animal protein. The main fats I ate were in seeds, nuts, and avocados. And I got all my protein from vegetable sources.

"Well, by the fifth day of the fast at least half of my pain had gone. The Hygienist doctor told me I must gradually lose weight and that a diet of fresh, living natural foods would restore my health to normal.

"Week by week, I gradually lost weight without dieting or feeling hungry. In eight weeks time, just as my weight reached normal, the last of the arthritis symptoms vanished.

"Since then, I've strictly avoided all fats, refined foods, and animal protein and monitored my fat intake. The arthritis never came back. And that hygienic diet of living foods is so zestful and revitalizing that, every year since, I've reached a new high plateau of health and wellness."

You Are Special

There is no one-diet-fits-all. The suggestions made in this book are meant to get you started on the highway to health and toward an arthritis-free existence.

But human beings are complex creatures, each with his own likes and dislikes, temperament, and physical peculiarities. This includes nutritional needs.

It's true that whole, unprocessed, chemical-free foods eaten in a serene atmosphere are best for everyone. It is equally true that many studies find vegetarians often bypass typical American diseases like osteoporosis, arthritis, and heart disease. Yet some people do better when they include some meat, dairy or eggs in their diet.

Joyce, a dedicated vegan for eight years, was tired and unenthusiastic at 35. Her naturopathic doctor suggested that one meat meal per week may alleviate her fatigue. Reluctant at first, Joyce ignored his advice. But daily fatigue finally convinced her to eat a steak; the results were dramatic.

"I found eating a little bit of meat made me feel stronger," reports Joyce. "Since then I eat one red meat dish each week—range fed and free of chemicals, of course."

As nutritional knowledge expands, we are learning that metabolic differences and ethnic background determine individual nutritional needs. For instance, if your grandparents immigrated from Scandinavia, you'll probably thrive on a fish-filled diet because you possess the genes of a people who've eaten fish for centuries. Likewise someone of Asian ancestry will most likely do well on rice.

Some people require a little animal protein for good health, for others this is a stressor food. Know your own needs by listening to what your symptoms and body are telling you. If meat makes your knees ache and plugs up your bowels, it's probably not for you. But if an occasional pork chop energizes you without adverse effects, you're probably destined to be a meat eater.

Learning to Recognize Stressor Foods

How do we recognize a stressor food? To do so, we must learn a few simple facts concerning nutrition. Fats, proteins, and carbohydrates are the main nutrients that comprise foods. Some foods are higher in one nutrient, say fat, than another; so we say they are a "fat." Meat is said to be a "protein", but contains fat too.

Fats are often divided into two main classes:

Saturated Fats: are so called because each of their carbon atoms are saturated with all the hydrogen they can hold. Saturated fats are hard or solid at room temperature, and primarily of animal origin (tropical oils like palm, palm kernel, and coconut are exceptions). We speak of fats as being either saturated or unsaturated; in reality fat composition is not an either-or situation. Both plant and animal fats contain *both* saturated and unsaturated portions (some even embody naturally occurring trans fatty acids). The difference being more animal foods are top heavy in saturated fats, while plants favor unsaturated oils. Some foods rich in saturated fats are high grade meats, organ meats, egg yolks, shell-fish, whole milk and dairy products, lard, and poultry skin.

Unsaturated Fats: have room to absorb more hydrogen atoms. They are liquid at room temperature and mainly of vegetable origin. Within the unsaturated fat category are two distinct classes. Polyunsaturated fats hold several (poly means many) openings for hydrogen atoms. Monounsaturated fats are crooked molecules with one (mono) double bond between two carbon atoms thus two hydrogen vacancies. Typical polyunsaturated fats are vegetable oils like safflower, soybean, sunflower, sesame, and corn oils. Macadamia oil, canola oil, and olive oil contain plenty of monounsaturated fats, and are thus considered monounsaturated oils. While liquid at room temperature, these oils tend to solidify in the fridge.

Cholesterol

Cholesterol is a fat-like substance called a sterol. Its notorious reputation is undeserved as the body relies on this sterol to build nerves, cell membranes, bile acids, and hormones. Cholesterol is only found in animal foods—meat, dairy, and eggs—and usually occurs alongside saturated fats.

Cholesterol is also synthesized by the liver in amounts often higher than what we typically eat each day. However, the body-made cholesterol is usually the high density lipoprotein (HDL) fraction—the type of cholesterol that does not cause heart disease. The low density lipoprotein (LDL) fraction, found primarily in foods, is responsible for hardening arteries and heart disease.

Atherosclerosis, or hardening of the arteries, is caused when cholesterol is deposited in the arteries like rust in a waterpipe, gradually blocking off oxygen and other essential nutrients to joints, heart, brain, and other organs. The result is weakened joints together with severe risk of heart attack, stroke, or hypertension. Artery and heart disease are also associated with high saturated fat intake.

Monounsaturated fats do not harm arteries or raise blood fat levels. These fats also help create the high density lipoprotein fraction of cholesterol that prevents LDL-cholesterol from clogging arteries.

On the other hand, eating a lot of polyunsaturated oils may lower helpful HDL-cholesterol. Polyunsaturated oils tend to turn rancid faster than monounsaturated oils. Rancid fats are one source of arthritis-provoking free radical molecules[44].

When compared to saturated fats which distort body chemistry, cause atherosclerosis, and aggravate arthritis and various diseases, unsaturated fats are not only harmless but help fight arthritis pain and inflammation.

Processing Makes Safe Foods Dangerous

But—and wouldn't you know it—the food processing industry has found a way to make these healthful vegetable oils highly dangerous. They have discovered how to inject these oils with more hydrogen atoms to turn them into trans fatty acids that are hard and solid at room temperature, just like saturated fats.

Be warned: these hydrogenated, or partially-hydrogenated vegetable oils are more dangerous than saturated fats. While low amounts of trans-fatty acids do occur naturally in beef and dairy products, consumption of these harmful fats didn't climb until after the 1897 invention of hydrogenation. These fats are widely used in margarine, factory breads, salad oils, mayonnaise, snack foods, and just about all processed foods. Ironically during the last 20 years Americans have switched in droves to cholesterol-free (trans-fatty acid-full) margarine, in the mistaken search for better health. In truth, trans fatty acids boost offensive LDL and total blood cholesterol, and drag down HDL[45].

A recent University of Maryland study that correlated fats in the human diet with increased risk of cancer made special mention of the extra hazards of partially-hydrogenated vegetable oils. Oils are hydrogenated to give them longer shelf life and to make them more profitable to the manufacturer. In doing so, of course, they shorten millions of human lives.

This isn't to say you should go overboard on plain vegetable oils either. Supermarket brands are usually brimming with chemicals used to extract the oils from nuts, seeds, and other fatty vegetable sources. Cold-pressed, freshly squeezed oils are a safer choice and are full of healthful, arthritis-fighting ingredients.

To prevent rancidity, store your oils in the fridge away from heat, light, and air. This precaution slows down oxidation and formation of hurtful free radical molecules that contribute to aging, cancer, and arthritis. Squeezing a capsule or two of the antioxidant nutrient, vitamin E, into your oil bottle every month will also delay rancidity. When cooking with vegetable oils, be careful not to heat them to the smoking point.

Another ideal way to eat healthy, anti-inflammatory oils is to simply eat the seeds, nuts, soybeans, and avocados from which vegetable oils are made. Remember, it's always best to eat food in it's original, whole form.

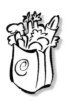

Dr. Hudson's Secret Seed Remedy

In Portland, Oregon, Dr. Tori Hudson, a noted natural health researcher, tells her arthritis patients to crush flax seeds in a coffee grinder or blender and spoon the healing meal on foods. "The anti-inflammatory quality of flax seeds is phenomenal," reports Dr. Hudson. Flax seed oil is even better, she says, and can be used as a salad dressing or mixed with low or non-fat cottage cheese as a super snack.

"Edgar Cayce, a renowned lay healer of long ago, suggested rubbing peanut oil into arthritic joints," Hudson adds. "I've had patients, a number of people in fact, who've told me this treatment really helps."

Stored-up Food Poisons May Spark Arthritic Disease

Saturated fats carry an extra danger signal. All animal fats have a proclivity for storing toxic petrochemicals, drugs used in animal feeds, and other poisons. The greater the fat content of any animal food, the greater the residue of chemical pesticides, insecticides, herbicides, and fertilizers stored in it. The higher up the food chain, the greater the risk. Many fruits and vegetables are sprayed as many as a dozen times before harvesting. When eaten by animals, poultry or fish, the pesticides on these plants become concentrated in an animal's tissues at 13 times the original level in the plant.

When an osprey, pelican, or eagle eats a fish in a river or estuary, the concentration of chlorinated hydrocarbons in its tissues can reach such toxic levels that the birds can no longer reproduce. You can imagine how these deadly poisons unbalance our body chemistry.

This is why we recommend eating only deep ocean fish and not fish or seafood from polluted rivers, lakes, coastal waters, or estuaries. Almost all are contaminated by agricultural run-off and industrial pollutants.

You probably never thought of cod or haddock as wild game. But these deep-ocean fish are the least contaminated wild game readily available. If you've ever wondered why native peoples from the far north living in their native habitat do not get most degenerative diseases despite all the meat and fish they eat, the reason is that they eat only wild game. Compared to the lethally high fat content of commercially-raised cattle, wild game such as whales, seals, and caribou have a comparatively low saturated fat concentration. For most of us, cod and haddock are the closest we can get to eating wild game.

A Natural Aspirin-Free Way to Reduce Pain and Inflammation

Fat contains twice as many calories per weight as carbohydrates or protein so it's easy to boost calories over the top with fatty indulgence. Health magazines, news reports, and doctors warn us to throw out the fat or else. But there's more to the fat story.

Fat is a necessary nutrient, used by the body to store energy, cushion cells, absorb fat-soluble nutrients, and keep immune systems humming. Women who eliminate fat from their diets stop menstruating. Dry flaky skin results when fat intake drops too low. And *arthritis gets worse when you don't eat enough of the right kind of fat.*

Two families of essential fatty acids (EFA) are vital for body function—and they must be obtained from foods. Omega-6 fats, one brand of EFA, come from plant sources like vegetable oils, flax and other seeds, nuts, as well as herbs like evening primrose and borage. Fish (and some plants) provide the other family of EFAs called omega-3 fats. Most whole, healthsome foods contain at least a smidgen of EFA.

These EFAs push your body to produce anti-inflammatory hormone-like chemicals called prostaglandins. There are many kinds of prostaglandins made throughout the body, but it's the series one and series three types that soothe painful, swollen joints. The series two prostaglandins, however, are pro-inflammatory, arthritis aching devils.

Peter Callegari, MD and his colleague Dr. Robert B. Zurier from the University of Pennsylvania in Philadelphia, outline in *Nutrition and Rheumatic Diseases* (1991, volume 17) the advantages of administering omega-6 EFAs to patients with rheumatoid arthritis. In various studies, primrose seed oil and borage seed oil both diminish swollen and tender joints to the point where pain pills are at least reduced. Gamma linolenic acid, called GLA for short, is a key omega-6 ingredient and arthritis healer found in these natural oils[46].

For decades, naturally-oriented practitioners, armed with this biochemical insight, have used these same remedies, and adjusted diet and other lifestyle habits to shunt prostaglandin production to the favorable, anti-inflammatory side. Saturated fat, hydrogenated oils and alcohol create painful series two prostaglandins, and swelling.

You can gently persuade prostaglandins to the painless side with omega-6 foods and the eicosapentanoic acid (EPA) of omega-3 oils found in salmon, mackerel, and other fatty fish. Ninety patients enrolled in a double-blind, randomized study in Belgium significantly improved after taking 2.6 grams of omega-3 fatty acids for one year, as one example[47].

While fatty fish are a must for healing arthritis, many fish are prohibited for those with gout because of their high purine and protein levels. However, pills containing EPA without other gout-provoking factors can be used. Most health food stores carry these supplements[48].

Foods rich in zinc, magnesium, and vitamins B6 and C, and niacin hurry the good prostaglandin stream along. Aging slows this process perhaps explaining why arthritis tends to be an illness of maturity.

Interestingly, aspirin and NSAID drugs work much the same as these miracle oils—by inhibiting inflammation-prone prostaglandins.

Protein

Protein provides building blocks for cells and tissue. It can be broken down into 22 different amino acids of which the body can synthesize only 14. The remaining eight (some nutritionists say 10) are called essential amino acids and must be obtained directly from foods. Virtually all animal-derived foods (including fish, poultry, dairy products, and eggs) contain whole protein which includes the eight essential amino acids.

Protein can also be supplied by vegetables, grains, nuts, and seeds. But no single plant-based food supplies whole protein. Vegetarians complement one protein-containing food with two or three others to obtain all eight essential amino acids.

We once thought plant proteins had to be eaten together to produce whole protein. It's now accepted that essential amino acids can be scattered throughout the day's meals. A well balanced, varied vegetarian diet consisting of grains, legumes, beans, fruits, and vegetables more than meets daily protein requirements.

The problem with animal protein is that you can easily eat too much, thereby creating four arthritis aggravating effects. First, excessive protein intake creates an imbalance in carbohydrate metabolism. Second, it may increase the amount of protein food particles in the bloodstream. Protein fragments are more likely to be recognized as foreign antigens than other types of foods.

Third, with few exceptions, to eat animal protein such as steak or liver, you must eat the high-fat content that comes along with it. And fourth, studies have shown that a high-protein diet may cause bone loss at twice the normal rate. Since calcium deficiency is a problem in some arthritis types, anything which accelerates bone loss is extremely undesirable.

The body's actual requirements for protein are amazingly small. A 160 pound man needs only 2 1/2 ounces of whole protein daily. Hence many nutritionists recommend that we derive a maximum of 15 percent of our calories from protein.

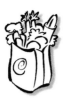

Carbohydrates

Carbohydrates are found in almost all fruits, vegetables, beans, legumes, and grains and are our main source of energy. Carbohydrates still carry the stigma of being fattening.

Not so! There are good and bad carbohydrates. And good carbohydrates—even those containing starch—are far from fattening.

The Good Carbohydrates

Good carbohydrates, called *complex, unrefined carbohydrates,* reside in whole, fresh fruits, vegetables, and grains as they come off the tree or out of the ground. Complex carbohydrates are found in all living foods (including nuts and seeds) that, if these foods were planted in the ground, they would grow into a plant or tree.

They are called complex because the living cells of these foods are encased in walls of cellulose. Cellulose and other components of fiber such as pectin cannot be digested by humans. They pass through the digestive system as fiber. All complex carbohydrate foods are also high in fiber.

Because fiber cannot be digested, the cell walls of complex carbohydrates decompose slowly, allowing the carbohydrates inside to enter the bloodstream at a slow, gradual pace without upsetting the pancreas' production and quality of insulin.

The Bad Carbohydrates

Bad carbohydrates are called *simple, refined carbohydrates*. They were originally complex carbohydrates, such as whole wheat berries that have been highly refined during milling. In refining, both the kernel and most grain fiber, vitamins, minerals, and enzymes are destroyed leaving little but the hollow calories and minimal nutrition of white flour.

Without fiber, refined carbohydrates are rapidly absorbed into the bloodstream. The sudden flush of sugar into which they are converted sends blood triglycerides and blood sugar levels soaring. Many heart specialists believe refined carbohydrates are as threatening to patients with heart disease as saturated fats or hydrogenated vegetable oils. The most common refined carbohydrate foods are sugar, white flour, and white rice.

Most natural nutritionists believe that 65 percent of our calories should come from complex carbohydrates and none at all from simple, refined carbohydrates. Several nutritionists have suggested that simple, refined carbohydrates are so menacing to health they should carry a warning sign like cigarettes.

The Stressor Foods
That Block the Healing
of Arthritis

All stressor foods are dead foods. If you planted them in the ground, they would *not* grow into living plants. These lifeless foods have another common drawback. They are sadly lacking in enzymes.

Enzymes are health promoting food components that in fresh, living foods aid digestion by acting as catalysts during food break-down. When dead foods are eaten, more digestive enzymes must be produced by the pancreas and other digestive organs. This stressful task taxes the body and lays the groundwork for arthritic disease.

Most canned, packaged, preserved, processed, manufactured, and convenience foods are dead and lifeless with much of their health restoring enzymes destroyed and most of the vitamin and mineral content depleted. Many frozen foods are also partially pre-cooked and are nutritionally empty and hollow.

Many foods are processed simply to give them longer shelf life. Yet no thought is ever given to extending the life of the consumer. Most processed foods are stressor foods and should be ruthlessly discarded from the diet.

177

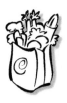

Pseudo Foods—A Travesty of Real Foods

Good health-promoting foods seldom come in boxes, packages, jars or cans. Nor are they cut up ahead of time or fragmented in any way. The only wholesome potatoes are whole potatoes in exactly the same state as they were dug from the ground with their skins intact and with sprouts budding out to prove they are still alive and have not been sprayed. Potatoes that are not whole are pseudo foods: instant mashed potatoes, French fries, potato chips, hashed browns, you name it—all are nutritional disasters guaranteed to hasten arthritis and other diseases.

Many foods which are not whole, fresh, raw, and completely natural are stressor foods. Any food that has been extensively processed or refined or that has been tampered with while growing is a stressor food.

Not all processed foods are bad. For instance bread made exclusively of 100 percent whole grain flour and entirely free of chemical additives is healthy food. Tofu is another example. These we'll try to point out as we go along.

How to Stop Committing Supermarket Suicide

Don't be misled into thinking that refined foods are okay after they've been fortified or enriched. Manufacturers may replace a few of the vitamins and minerals they've destroyed in refining. But the foods are still devoid of most enzymes and fiber.

Supermarket shelves abound with boxes and packages of counterfeit foods which bear long lists of the many vitamins and minerals they contain. The lists may sound impressive, but the foods still contain chemical preservatives and artificial coloring or flavor. And their fiber content is often completely devitalized.

Don't be fooled by containers which state "no artificial anything." Actually, the manufacturer is telling the truth. All the emulsifiers, anti-bacterial agents, bleaches, blenders, anti-caking, and anti-fungal agents that some foods contain are not artificial. They are real, honest-to-goodness chemical additives.

Take a cold, hard look at any food container labeled "All natural ingredients" or "No artificial preservatives added." These terms, especially natural, are often misused by manufacturers. Read labels to see what's *really* in that food you're eating. The most wholesome, health building foods rarely come in boxes, cans, jars, or packages.

Most jars of jam or preserves labeled "no artificial preservatives" state the literal truth. What they don't tell you is that the high sugar content of the fruit itself preserves the jam. In doing so, it counteracts the nutritional goodness of the fruit.

Other than freezing, in which absolutely no chemicals are used, drying is the best way to preserve foods. Even that is second choice.

In drying, foods like dates, figs, and raisins are concentrated versions of already sweet fruit. When eaten, they produce the same flush of sugar in the bloodstream as do refined carbohydrates. A few dried fruits can be safely eaten from time to time. Small amounts of raisins mixed with nuts or seeds, or used for similar flavoring, can be eaten daily. But frequent binges of dried fruits in large amounts is another nutritional no-no.

To sum up: The food processing industry created the modern western diet. As this devitalized diet was adopted, the incidence of heart disease, colon and breast cancer, diabetes, osteoporosis, and arthritis all increased right in step.

Just because everyone else goes on eating this harmful western diet, you don't have to.

To avoid it, totally ignore the row upon row of cans, boxes, jars, and packaged foods that line your supermarket shelves. Shop instead in the produce section or patronize your local natural health markets. By cutting out dead foods from your diet and replacing them with fresh, living foods, you can transform your present harmful, modern diet into the same health-building, primitive diet on which the human body has thrived for millennia.

Rebecca S. Discovers That Arthritis Is the Junk Food Disease

It was difficult to believe that the tireless, radiantly healthy woman who enjoys a thorough trouncing on the tennis court was crippled with arthritis until eight years ago.

"The pain first appeared in my back and ribs when I was 54," Rebecca S. said after the game. "I visited a number of doctors. None could do anything. In the end I spent a week at a diagnostic clinic. They said I had osteoarthritis of the spine and that it was incurable.

"From then on life became an endless round of aspirin and constant, miserable pain. I still can't believe that I put up with that constant agony for three whole years.

"No one at the clinic told me that being overweight was half the cause. Or that all the fat and sugar I was eating had any effect on arthritis. At last, a friend suggested I see an herbalist.

"Well, the herbalist, a very knowledgeable German lady, said I was too far gone for herbs to help much. She said if I were ever to get well I'd better decide to help myself right now. She told me about treating disease with food.

"She said I must stop eating dead foods like sugar and refined flour as well as foods of animal origin, and stimulants. I was to eat nothing but fresh, natural living foods instead.

"The pain and aspirin had me so frustrated I was ready to clutch at anything. I followed her advice exactly.

"Slowly, a bit at a time, I did begin to feel better. After six weeks, I lost 12 pounds and the pain in my back was definitely fading. I could walk and do housework again.

"I had to lose 18 more pounds before the pain ended. My back was still filled with calcium deposits. Every time I moved, my back cracked and groaned. The German lady taught me yoga bending exercises. Every day I'd bend my spine easily and gently in every direction. Eventually, my spine limbered up.

"But I'd still have an occasional flare-up. The lady tested my pulse and found I was allergic to corn, potatoes, and tomatoes. As soon as I dropped these foods, the flare-ups stopped coming back.

"Now I can walk five miles, swim for an hour, or play tennis half the day. I do eat some corn, potatoes, and tomatoes on a rotational basis once a week. But I never eat anything that contains lots of fat, refined foods, alcohol or caffeine. All my friends still eat these lifeless foods. But I'm the only one who is completely healthy and free of any chronic disease."

Stressor Foods You Should Never Eat Again

Here, as a guide to what foods to avoid, is a brief run down.

ALCOHOL: While a moderate amount of alcohol increases the good HDL cholesterol, there are much safer ways to alter cholesterol levels. Alcohol depletes the body's supply of B-vitamins and paves the way for arthritis by interfering with body functions.

CAFFEINE is a legal shot of speed that creates a high by distorting the output of adrenal—an essential body gland. Whether in coffee, cocoa, chocolate, some soft drinks, or black tea, caffeine is a highly addictive food that invariably tests allergy positive. Caffeine is also a vitamin antagonist and is often taken with sugar, another stressor food.

You can easily overcome its addiction by each day replacing one cup of coffee with a cup of tea. Black tea has half the caffeine content of coffee. If your daily quota is seven cups of coffee, in one week you can replace it with seven cups of tea and cut your caffeine intake by half. The following week, replace one cup of tea per day with a cup of herbal tea or carob. In 14 days, you will have overcome the caffeine habit completely.

CHEMICAL ADDITIVES: Anyone who eats the conventional American way takes 4–5 pounds of chemical additives into the body each year. Despite the banning of a few dyes and other dangerous additives by the FDA, at least 3,000 additives remain in use—and are increasing every year.

The majority have not been tested for safety by the FDA. Their safety is determined by the food processing industry itself, often in laboratories subsidized by the manufacturers. Stored in body fat, these poisons hasten arthritis by interfering with or disrupting body functions. Many are also known to cause cancer.

Some brands of ice cream and diet sodas may contain 50 percent of chemical additives. Almost every processed food carries a host of nitrites, coloring, stabilizers, bleaching agents, texturing agents, emulsifiers, or other chemicals, few of which have ever been tested for their long-term danger to human life. Texturing agents make limp canned vegetables appear crisp and fresh. Flavoring agents mask a disagreeable taste. Even a wholesome food like yogurt often contains stressor foods like sugar and artificial fruit flavors.

CONDIMENTS per se are not evil foods. In fact many traditional healing systems revere spices for their curative effects. The thousands of years old Ayurvedic medical system embraces strong spices like turmeric as digestive aids. Allspice, cumin, basil, oregano, and star anise are traditional arthritis remedies in the herbal world. (See Chapter 14 for more on these helpful spices.)

Undoubtedly, some condiments should be avoided. Commercial sauces like ketchup and salad dressings are full of sugar and additives. Salt, another favorite additive and condiment, can cause arthritis symptoms by creating edema in joints.

The worst condiment is (MSG) mono-sodium glutamate widely used in cooking at cafeterias and Chinese restaurants to supposedly enhance taste. After eating MSG-doped food, thousands of people have discovered the MSG syndrome—headaches, stiffness in the neck, jaw, and other joints, and numbness in the limbs.

By all means throw out all these foodless foods. But keep the spice in your life—it may even help your arthritis.

COW'S MILK is fine for calves. But millions of children and adults are unable to tolerate the lactose, fat or protein in milk. Many older people cannot absorb the calcium in milk, a problem that may lead to osteoporosis or arthritis, if dairy is your main calcium source. The same intolerance may extend to dairy products like cream or cheese. Seventy percent of African-Americans have difficulty digesting milk. Cow's milk and its products are also a major arthritis provoking allergen.

However, if you have no sensitivity to dairy, non-fat cottage cheese or non-fat yogurt, when entirely free of other stressor foods or additives, are sound health restoring foods.

SUGAR is present in almost all processed foods. Most Americans consume two pounds or more of this stressful food each week. Sugar causes the blood sugar level to soar. Then just as suddenly, it plummets and lets you down. In doing so, it upsets both the pancreas and the action of the adrenal glands. Eating sugar suppresses the immune system, opening the way for arthritis and other diseases.

Most brown sugar is simply white sugar coated with molasses, while turbanide sugar is partially refined. Not recommended is aspartame or any other synthetic sweetener. Nor is extracted fructose recommended as a sugar substitute.

The best sweetener is no sweetener at all. However, if you must have a substitute, blackstrap molasses is the best alternative. It is rich in B-vitamins, iron, and other minerals. Honey or maple syrup that is raw, unfiltered, and unheated can also be used in small amounts in place of sugar.

Even though nutritionally more desirable than refined sugar, these sweeteners can have the same effect on body chemistry. If you must have something sweet, try a few dates, figs, or raisins, some sweet, fresh fruits, or sweet vegetables like baked yams or carrots.

While freshly squeezed fruit juice is better than canned or frozen and is superior to soda, it's still concentrated sugar. Dilute all fruit juices half and half with pure water. Better yet, quench your thirst with water alone.

Pain Folds its Fangs when Ella C. Stops Eating Stressor Foods

Can you imagine anyone being grateful for having a heart attack?

Ella C. is. At 58, Ella began suffering with osteoarthritis pain in the hips and knees.

But hear her story in her own words.

"I was overweight and the pain in my hips was so severe that only a shot of Novocain™ could bring relief. My rheumatologist said it was progressive and at my age would never improve.

"My diet was full of fat, and I snacked on sugar filled foods all day. Yet I was never advised to change my diet.

"The following year I had a heart attack. Fortunately it was just a mild one. As a result, I came under the care of a cardiologist. He was appalled at my diet.

"He cut out all of the fat, sugar, and high fat meats, and dairy I loved. He said if I didn't stick to the diet I'd have another heart attack soon and this one would be fatal.

"As you can imagine, I stuck right with that diet. Instead of the fat and sugar, I ate fresh fruit and vegetable salads. I soon came to love the honest taste of these living foods and I used no artificial condiments at all.

"It took three months for my weight to drop back to normal. Every week, as my weight went down, my arthritis also began to disappear. On the day my weight reached normal, the last of my arthritis symptoms vanished.

"The cardiologist said mine was one of several cases he'd seen where a person had changed their diet to recover from heart disease and then found that the same diet brought recovery from arthritis.

"He said that the cholesterol that was clogging the arteries to my heart also blocked the flow of blood and nutrients to my knees and hips.

"When I got rid of the cause of arthritis, the saturated fat and sugar, and other junk that made me overweight and clogged my arteries, my body healed itself. But if I'd never had the heart attack, I'd still be suffering with arthritis today."

Ella C. is now a hale and hearty 68 and has been totally free of both arthritis and heart disease symptoms for more than eight years.

 Profile of Peril—The Worst Foods You Can Eat

This is a nearly complete list of all stressor foods and Stressor ingredients that cause nutritional distress and that can lead, eventually, to arthritis, and other degenerative diseases. Whether or not you have arthritis, to attain optimum health all should be totally excluded from your diet on a lifelong basis. The list is in addition to other stressor foods already mentioned in this chapter.

The list refers only to commercial products. Health food stores often carry more acceptable forms of some foods. Too, some of these foods can be prepared at home with more wholesome ingredients.

Additives

Alcohol

Artificial dairy foods

Artificial sweeteners

Aspartame

Bacon (*fatty, strip*)

Bakery products

Beef tallowMargarine

BeerMarmalade

Bouillon cubes

Bread (*commercial*)

Breakfast cereals (*containing sugar*)

Broth (*canned*)

Brown sugar

Butter

Cakes

Cake mixes

CandyPastry

Canned foods

Chinese food (*high fat—restaurant variety*)

Chocolate

Coffee

Cola drinks

Convenience foods

Crackers

Cream

Dairy foods (*whole fat*)

Dairy substitutes

Diet sodas and colas

Doughnuts

Dry drink powders

Fast foods

Fatty meats

Flour (*refined, bleached, enriched*)

French fries

Fried foods

Fried rice

Frozen desserts

Frozen dinners

Frozen pre-cooked foods

Frozen yogurt

Gravies

Honey (*processed*)

Hot dogs

Hydrogenated or partially hydrogenated vegetable oils

Ice cream (*whole fat*)

Ice milk

Instant breakfasts

Instant foods (*all types*)

Jams

Jellies

Jello

Ketchup

Lard

Liquor

Luncheon meats

Mayonnaise

Meat (*red, fatty*)

Milk (*homogenized whole cow's milk*)

Monosodium glutamate (MSG)

Nitrates, nitrites

Non-dairy creamers

Noodles (*refined*)

Pasta (*refined*)

Potatoes (*flakes, chips, processed*)

Poultry skin

Powdered whole milk

Prepared mixes

Pre-prepared main dishes, desserts, etc.

Preserves

Puddings

Pudding mixes

Quick-preparation foods (*all types*)

Rice (*refined, hulled*)

Saccharine

Salad dressings

Salt

Sausage

Sherbert

Shortening

Smoked foods

Soft drinks

Soup

Sour cream (*whole fat*)

Spaghetti (*refined*)

Spare ribs (*fatty*)

Suet

Sugar

Tea (*black*)

Tobacco smoke

Turbanide sugar

TV dinners

White bread

White flour

White rice

Wine

You'll notice we didn't place eggs, all dairy foods, or all meats on the stressor list. That's because some of you will do fine eating low fat versions of these foods in moderation. Just remember the Asian and Mediterranean food pyramids where animal proteins are treated as condiments, not everyday or main dishes.

To make this nutrition lesson even more complex, did you know that scientists are discovering that not all saturated fats are as bad as originally thought? Stearic acid, one component of some saturated fats, has less cholesterol raising abilities than other constituents.

The Semi-Stressor Foods

Now add to the above list semi-stressor foods, items that have been sprayed with pesticides, grown in soils replete with synthetic fertilizers or covered in other chemicals. Irradiated foods fit into this category, and possibly genetically engineered foods. Animal products that have been shot up with antibiotics, hormones, or other chemicals may also be included.

Although there's no doubt these foods hurt health, in many cases its impossible to find chemical-free, pure plant, or animal foods. So rather than demand you avoid these foods totally (and perhaps starve to death), we delegate these items to the semi-stressor category. It's more important that you consume an abundance of fresh fruits and vegetables than not.

We strongly encourage you to seek out vendors and farmers dedicated to organic farming and ranching. Buy their wares not only for your overall health, but to ensure that these high quality foods will continue to be available to everyone.

Cutting Out Stressor Foods Ends John L.'s Nagging Gout

"I was racked with constant, throbbing pain," is how 53-year-old John L. described his gout. "My toes and insteps were excruciatingly tender, and the flesh over the joints had turned hard, shiny, and purple.

"My doctor told me it was caused by purines in certain foods. He said it was easier to control gout with drugs than to bother going on a diet. But the drugs gave me itchy skin, headaches, abdominal pain, and diarrhea. For me, the cure was as bad as the disease.

"Finally, I went to a nutritionist. He put me on a five-day water fast. Then I had to cut out all foods that contained purines.

"In just two weeks, the pain and inflammation in my joints subsided. But I still continued to have minor flare-ups. The nutritionist said these are due to my being overweight. He said that if I dropped my weight back to normal they would disappear."

John L. did eventually lose weight, and the rest of his gout disappeared along with the surplus pounds.

As John L. discovered, many doctors today treat gout with drugs instead of diet. The reason given is that patients will usually not stick to their diet. Also most gout sufferers are overweight. To become completely gout-free, weight must be reduced to normal.

Forbidden Foods for Those with Gout

Gout is aggravated by an excess of purines in the diet. Purines are the basic substance of uric acid. They abound in such rich foods as organ meats, goose, and caviar. Other oily, fatty delicacies reduce uric acid excretion, as does excessive protein. Alcohol is eliminated from a gout diet because it may increase uric acid production. Coffee and sugar aren't known to affect gout directly, but should be avoided for overall health reasons.

Until purine-rich and fatty foods are totally eliminated from the diet, gout cannot be reversed. Here is a list of the gout-provoking foods that John L. was forbidden to eat:

Alcohol	Mackerel
Anchovies	Meat soup
Beef tongue	Mussels
Bouillon	Organ meats
Brains	Oysters
Caviar	*Pork
*Clams	Sardines
Coffee	Sausage
Consommé	Scrabble
Duck	*Shellfish
Fish roe	*Shrimp
Goose	Soft drinks
Gravies	Squab
Herring	Sugar
Kidneys	Sweetbreads
Liver	Yeast

Foods with an asterisk contain moderate amounts of purines and may be consumed occasionally. It's impossible to avoid purines altogether; the goal is to keep your levels down. So to keep your case of gout under control, it is absolutely vital to eliminate every non-asterisked food totally, immediately, and for always. Right after that, cut out all of the stressor foods.

How to Immunize Yourself Against Gout, Arthritis, and All Killer Diseases

Regardless of what type of arthritic disease you have—or even if you do not have arthritic disease—you should strictly avoid all stressor foods *for the rest of your life*. These life-threatening foods pave the way for *all* types of degenerative disease, not merely gout or arthritis.

Eliminate these foods entirely and you will have drastically immunized yourself against not only gout or arthritis but also heart disease, hypertension, diabetes, osteoporosis, diverticulosis, kidney disease, and other killer diseases that flourish wherever the western diet has appeared.

Chapter **12**

The Incredible Arthritis-Healing Powers of Restorative Foods

The body heals itself when the *cause* of disease is removed. This is the natural law of healing.

We have removed the aggravators of arthritic disease—the stressor foods that stress the joints with overweight and poor nutrition and the allergy foods which trigger the immune system to harass cells in weakened joints. Not least of all, we have healed the digestive tract, the body's life line.

But let's always remember that arthritis is nothing more than the body's way of responding to this stress and attack. The pain, stiffness, and inflammation of arthritis are all responses by the body as it attempts to defend itself.

The body itself creates gout and arthritis. Therefore, the body itself can heal arthritis.

To do so, we have only to remove the offenders—the stressor and allergy foods—and to replace them with restorative foods that rebuild the ailing body and restore its biochemical balance.

Undoubtedly, after reading the list of stressor foods that are now forbidden, you are probably wondering what there is left to eat.

How about:

- *The entire vegetable kingdom*: that is, every single fruit, legume, vegetable, bean, and sprout in existence; also soybean products like tofu and tempeh.

- *The entire grain kingdom*: A whole spectrum of cereals and grains, provided they are unrefined, are: hardy, satisfying foods..

- *All nuts and seeds*. Nuts and seeds are rich in nutrients the body needs to heal itself. Non-rancid polyunsaturated, omega-6 nut and seed oils, used sparingly, decrease joint swelling.

- *Low-fat foods of animal origin* such as egg whites, lean meats, non-fat dairy foods, and skinless poultry.

- *Monounsaturated oils* such as olive and canola oils used sparingly provide omega-3 fatty acids that battle inflammation and the pain of arthritis.

- *Fatty fish* like salmon and herring, the best source of omega-3 fatty acids, are a regular must to ease inflammation and misery.

At any supermarket produce counter, you have a choice of at least 12 and up to 20 different vegetables and a dozen different fruits depending on season. Most supermarkets carry at least half a dozen varieties of dried beans as well as a choice of whole grains, dried fruits, and unsalted nuts.

Elsewhere in your supermarket you'll find frozen or fresh cold-water fish, lean meats like veal, and non-fat cheese and yogurt.

Health food stores are not just specialty shops anymore. If you live in a moderate size or large city, look for supermarkets that carry only healthy, natural, and organic foods. In some areas, these stores are run as cooperatives where for a small fee you become a member; many cooperatives allow non-members to shop also.

You'll find at least a dozen different unsprayed grains. Many carry up to 20 or more varieties together with a dozen different types of beans, eight or more varieties of nuts, several different seeds for eating, and a variety of seeds and grains for sprouting. These stores also carry breads made entirely from whole grains and free of hydrogenated oils and other destructive foods.

They stock low or non-fat organic dairy foods and raw milk. Range-fed ,chemical-free meats and poultry are a normal item. If you want to buy packaged foods, you can be assured that their soups, cereals, pastas, sauces, and everything else you normally find in a conventional supermarket (many listed in our book as stressor foods) will be here also—only, for the most part, made with wholesome ingredients and without harmful additives.

Finding Super Nutrition in Your Supermarket

In their whole, natural form exactly as they come from the tree, the ground, the animal or from the ocean, these restorative foods will supply your body with all the nutrients it needs to rebuild damaged joints and restore high-level wellness.

A very few exceptions like non-fat dairy foods and tofu have been mildly processed; beans, raisins, and dates have been dried; and meat and fish may have been frozen. But most other Restorative Foods are fresh and alive.

Even dried beans are alive, and yogurt contains living bacteria. Every fresh, raw fruit, vegetable, grain, nut, and seed is still living. All grains, nuts, seeds, and fruits, as well as vegetables like potatoes, will sprout and grow if planted in the ground. The cells in green, leafy vegetables continue to live until the leaves wilt and droop.

Dead foods make listless, lifeless people prone to disease. Many restorative foods are fresh and alive shortly before eating. The reason is that they are grown, not manufactured. All their health-building chlorophyll, vitamins, minerals, enzymes, and fiber are mainly intact.

The Natural Healing Values of Certain Common Fruits and Vegetables

Many of nature's restorative foods are so commonplace that their nutritional healing values have been overlooked. But all vegetables, fruits, grains, nuts, and seeds are natural foods that work to bring about positive changes in both mind and body. And to ensure total health, nutrition must be viewed in terms of the whole person rather than in terms of trying to cure a specific disease.

So let's not underestimate the value of whole, simple, natural foods. Some very plain-jane fruits and vegetables are making news in scientific circles for their healing and protective qualities. And if natural foods hadn't made so many people feel better, they would never have achieved their present popularity.

Guidelines for Eating Away Arthritis

- Buy and eat as many whole, fresh, raw, still-living foods as possible in their natural, unprocessed state free of salt and additives. This means buying fresh, raw fruits and vegetables, whole grains, and whole nuts and seeds—unchanged in any way by man and exactly as nature produced them. Shop organic when you can.

- Eat as many foods as possible uncooked or lightly steamed. If you chop up your food, do so just before serving. If you cannot chew raw vegetables, nuts, or seeds, then cut them up or grind them just before eating. But if your teeth are good, serve as many foods as possible whole and unfragmented. This way, they retain most of their enzymes, vitamins, and fiber.

- Avoid cooking any foods you can enjoy eating raw. If you must cook your vegetables, steam until crispy. Foods that must be cooked, like grains, potatoes, meat, fish, or dried beans, should be cooked only until done; avoid overcooking. This preserves their vitamins and some enzymes. Keep cooked dishes small and few and raw food dishes large and numerous.

- Follow the 65-20-15 formula. Combine your foods so that 65 percent or more of your calories are derived from complex carbohydrates, a maximum of 20 percent from fats, and 15 percent from protein.

- Eat at least twice as many vegetables as fruits. Vegetables are rich in chlorophyll, vitamins, minerals and fiber, and lower in sugar. (Note some dark colored fruits like cherries and berries provide valuable flavonoids for healing arthritis.)

- Before eating any cooked dish, eat a large salad of vegetables, including bitter lettuces, first. Or eat a large amount of raw vegetables with the cooked item. This will supply some of the enzymes, vitamins, and fiber that have been destroyed by cooking.

- Avoid eating fruits and vegetables (and other incompatible combinations) at the same meal.

- Eat foods that are in season and grown locally. This seasonal-regional principle comes to us from macrobiotic teachings, a healing way of eating and living.

- Get your fat from cold-pressed vegetable oils (canola and olive oils are preferable), nuts, seeds, avocados and plenty of omega-3 fatty fish. Add flax seed meal to your dishes for extra anti-inflammatory power.

- Obtain protein from plant sources or else from deep ocean fish, egg whites, very lean meat, or very low- or non-fat dairy foods.

- Eat as wide a variety of restorative foods as you can. Avoid eating the same foods every day.

We'll explain these guidelines as we go along. But first, we're sure you'd like to know what a typical meal of restorative foods looks and tastes like.

Dr. Donovan's Anti-Arthritis Diet Plan

At both of his clinics located in the beautiful Pacific Northwest, Dr. Patrick Donovan, a naturopathic physician who specializes in treating arthritis naturally, tells his patients to push stressor foods out of their diets with restorative foods.

He also has them follow the 3-S rule during mealtime: eat *several small simple* meals.

Digestion is endangered when we consume large amounts of poor quality foods in complex combinations. Using the 3-S rule and taking into account forbidden allergy foods, here is a sample of what Dr. Donovan recommends for a day's menu.

Breakfast: A fresh raw fruit salad containing apples, bananas, and pineapple. A heaping bowl of oatmeal with 1/2 cup of non-fat plain yogurt drizzled on top.

Snack: An assortment of vegetable sticks like jicama and celery are great mid-morning munchers.

Lunch: A large raw vegetable salad. For example, dark leafy lettuces, carrot, cucumber, bean sprouts, and a slice of avocado. Include a vegetable protein like baked pinto beans or lentil soup. Top it off with a side dish of grains, possibly brown rice or a slice of whole sprout bread.

Snack: A handful of dates and raw, unsalted almonds will carry you through to dinner.

Dinner: Start with a raw vegetable salad. Cook up fish or other selected animal protein (if animal foods disagree with you, substitute beans, legumes, or other high protein vegetable foods.) Millet or quinoa make nice grain entrees.

Snack: A fresh peach, plum, or other raw fruit makes a good before bedtime snack.

Dr. Donovan recommends making lunch the largest meal of the day. But in the name of practicality, he has designed the above menu plan with a large dinner in mind as most people eat their biggest meal in the evening with family or friends.

A Recipe for the Most Important Meal of the Day

If you find breakfast time to be extra hectic, prepare this delicious and nutritious drink and get to work on time.

The Frantic Fruit Smoothie

Toss the following ingredients into the blender:

3 or 4 different fruits including blueberries or cherries (frozen is okay if fresh is not available; don't use citrus fruit)

One Tbsp. flax seed meal or flax seed oil

1/2 cup non-fat yogurt

1/4 to 1/2 cup raw oatbran

Blend until smooth and enjoy. If you wish, you can make this smoothie the night before and store in the refrigerator.

Each Unto His Own

Nutritional guidelines are handy. But you must find your own personal, workable diet. A plant based, high fiber eating plan is encouraged along with cold water, omega-3 wealthy fish. But individual allergies, metabolic makeup, and ethnic idiosyncrasies should be woven into our recommendations to create a dietary program tailored to you.

Diet habits should also change with the seasons. During the spring and summer months, vegetables and fruits should hoover around a 75 percent high. Heavier foods like grains, legumes, seeds and nuts, and animal products comprise the rest of the diet. When the weather turns cold during autumn and winter, heavier protein and fat foods are desirable, while a mere 40 percent of the diet incorporates fruits and vegetables[49].

Natural Foods—The Fast, Convenient Way to Eat

Can natural foods be fast, convenient foods? Many restorative foods take less time to prepare than most conventional fast foods and less time to clean up afterwards.

Instead of tearing down your health, as do commercial fast foods, "fast convenience" living foods give you every nutrient your body needs to get better from arthritis and to stay well for life. Reach your optimum weight without paying any attention to calories.

You do not need to add bran to your food because almost every recommended item is high in fiber. Most of these foods supply extra enzymes for digestion. Every item is rich in vitamins and minerals. You get all the protein, fat, and carbohydrates your body requires. And you don't need to mask the taste with junk food sauce because natural foods provide a rich mixture of flavor nuances.

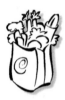

Natural Foods End Most Digestive Problems for Good

Aren't uncooked foods difficult to digest?

Although some starchy foods, along with cereals and beans, are easier to digest cooked, most fruits, vegetables, nuts, and seeds are easier to digest raw. The exception is anyone with inflammatory bowel disease.

The reason is that raw foods carry enzymes which our bodies use in digesting food. For example, the enzyme protease is used in digesting protein, lipase in digesting fats, and amylase in digesting carbohydrates. Cooking depletes foods of many enzymes used for digestion.

Most people who experience gas or indigestion after eating raw high fiber foods need only give themselves a few months to adjust. The friendly bacteria in your gut need time to settle down and get used to metabolizing all the wonderful fiber passing through your intestine now. Eating too much or too fast or consuming meals when your stomach is tight also creates bloating.

Some nutritionists and natural health practitioners think how you combine your foods affects digestion. Food combining is used therapeutically for degenerative diseases like arthritis and to repair digestion.

Food combining specialists classify foods into four categories: vegetables, fruits, proteins, and starches. Protein foods include nuts, beans, and seeds (as well, as all animal-derived foods). Starches include such starchy vegetables as yams, parsnips, and potatoes. Almost all foods in any one category are compatible with one another. But the different categories should be combined only like this:

GOOD COMBINATIONS

- Vegetables and starch foods
- Vegetables and protein foods

POOR COMBINATIONS

- Vegetables and fruits
- Proteins and fruits
- Starches and fruits
- Starches and proteins

Citrus fruits and melons often don't combine well with other foods and should be eaten alone.

The practice of food combining is dismissed by most mainstream nutritionists as folly. They say we have all the enzymes needed to break down any combination of foods simultaneously. And it is true, that as a science, food combining ranks poorly.

However, there is some scientific evidence to back up this approach. Several years ago, researchers found that when fat, especially the poorly absorbed, hydrogenated kind, and simple carbohydrates were eaten together with protein, stomach acid and digestive enzymes dropped. This set the scene for large, partially digested protein particles to pass from the gut into general circulation[35].

From a practical standpoint, different food types are broken down at different speeds. Thus combining foods with similar digestion times probably does give your gastrointestinal tract a break. Over the years, food combining advocates have noticed that patients with numerous food allergies or poor digestion do better when they eat simple meals and don't mix certain foods.

Like the other recommendations in this book, apply food combining principles only if they improve your symptoms and health. Listen to your body.

Only Living Foods Contain Anti-Arthritic Nutrients

Only raw foods have any appreciable nutritional value because cooking, processing, or storing destroys 50–70 percent of most vitamins. For example, canning or freezing can destroy up to 90 percent of a food's vitamin B_6 value. Processed foods and frozen juices have lost almost all of their vitamin C. Both B_6 and C are essential vitamins for reversing arthritis.

Cooking meats and vegetables destroys up to 85 percent of most vitamins. The nutrients that most of us think exist in cooked and processed foods actually don't. Nutritional research is showing that modern processed foods often contain 66 percent fewer vitamins than are listed for these foods in government nutrition handbooks.

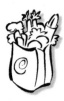

Living Foods End Both Colitis and Arthritis for Bernice W.

Bernice W. was 39 when she was diagnosed as suffering from ulcerative colitis. Her doctor placed her on a high-protein diet, high in saturated fats and low in fiber. Severe side effects prevented her doctor from using cortisone. But during the two following years, he prescribed no fewer than 14 different drugs, none of which produced the slightest benefit.

At age 42, Bernice was attacked by pains in her fingers, wrists, and left knee. The pains appeared quite suddenly with stiffness and inflammation following. Her doctor diagnosed the new ailment as rheumatoid arthritis, no doubt related to her intestinal troubles.

The two diseases combined turned Bernice into a bedridden invalid. Her colitis prevented Bernice from taking aspirin or any of the standard arthritis drugs. As a result, her doctor advised Bernice to have her colon removed and to move her bowels into a plastic bag hooked to her waist. She would then be able to take drugs for arthritis.

Bernice was shocked at the suggestion of a cure which would have turned her into a lifelong invalid. She turned to reading nutrition magazines. She learned of a natural hygiene health school located nearby, and the doctor in charge agreed to take her.

The hygienic doctor was horrified at Bernice's condition and her diet of protein and drugs. He found she was also suffering from osteoporosis, bone loss brought on by the high protein diet.

Although Bernice was slightly underweight, she was placed on a five-day fast. All drugs were withheld. At the end of the fourth day with neither food nor drugs, Bernice became aware that the pains in her joints had almost disappeared. For the first time in months, she got out of bed and walked. Her constant diarrhea also ended during the fast.

She was placed on a diet of fresh, raw fruits, vegetables, nuts, and seeds and told to stay with them for life. Bernice was amazed and delighted to watch both her colitis and arthritis gradually slip away. She took no more drugs. Within six weeks, she felt fully recovered.

Although doctors customarily place colitis patients on a diet of bland, cooked foods with lots of protein to "build up the body" Bernice experienced no difficulty at all in assimilating a diet of uncooked natural foods. The hygienic doctor explained that this was because all living foods that abound in enzymes are needed for digestion.

All this took place 20 years ago. Now a fit and youthful 63, Bernice has remained a food purist and has had no trace of either colitis or arthritis. Except for lightly baking potatoes and other starchy vegetables, her diet consists exclusively of fresh, living foods. (Please note, high fiber raw foods should be avoided during an acute flare-up of ulcerative colitis.)

How to Retain Nutrients While Cooking

To do the least harm to foods by cooking, cook as little as possible. Use as little water as you can, cook for the shortest time possible, and use the lowest temperature. Cooked foods should be crisp not waterlogged and soggy. Serve immediately.

Light baking is probably the least damaging way to cook followed by steaming, or sautéeing with water or canola oil. Almost any type of starchy vegetable tastes delicious when lightly baked. Try to undercook as far as possible, and always keep the lid on.

Beans and cereals can be lightly cooked in a pressure cooker or crock pot. This way, you can minimize loss of vitamins and enzymes while cooking.

Boiling or stewing is least desirable because most vitamins are water soluble and dissolve in the cooking water. If you do boil or steam, save the water and add to soups. Frying in lard, of course, is unthinkable.

You Can Continue to Eat Lots of Good Things

Bearing these principals in mind, there are still lots of good things you can continue to eat. Dozens of delicious, low-fat dishes can be made from corn, rice, and other whole grains. Many Mideastern Oriental and other ethnic dishes are low in fat and can be safely prepared at home without salt or MSG. Whole grain spaghetti and other types of pasta are sold in health food stores and many supermarkets and are superior to the white, enriched brands.

Tempting soups can be prepared from vegetables, beans, or fruit and thickened with brown rice. For example, potato, cauliflower, onion, cabbage, tomato, celery, lentil, soybeans, and white beans are all good in soups. Add turmeric, cayenne or other healing spices described in Chapter 14. Because you don't throw away the cooking water, soups retain most vitamins. Whole grain breads, pita bread, and corn tortillas go well with soups.

For sweet tasting vegetables, try a mix of lightly baked yams, parsnips, and carrots with parsley. Adding onions, parsley, bay leaf, and garlic to soups and cooked dishes adds spice to the taste.

Parsley is rich in vitamin A and other nutrients which arthritis sufferers often lack. To richen taste, blend foods with a mixture of raw tomatoes, cucumbers, and avocados.

For a salad dressing, try one of the cold-pressed oils described earlier under "fats", or use a non-fat plain yogurt or cottage cheese.

You can eat eggs safely by simply hardboiling them, then removing the yolk and eating only the white part. Or try a cholesterol-free omelette made of egg whites with sliced green onions and chopped parsley served on a slice of whole grain bread or toast. And, of course, literally scores of tasty dishes can be made by combining fish with vegetables and grains. Very lean meat and skinless poultry can be alternated with fish for greater variety.

Desserts? Although it's wisest not to mix fruits with other types of foods, if you wait a short time after a meal, you can safely serve stewed prunes, a few dates and figs, a dish of fresh, mixed fruit. Or freeze a whole peeled banana and see if you can taste the difference between it and ice cream. Freeze any fruit and put it through a juicer—it tastes delicious.

Convert your favorite cookie and loaf recipes into healthy, new ones. Substitute white flour with whole grain flours like barley or wheat. Use the whites of two eggs for every whole egg. Instead of lard or shortening, add applesauce and/or canola oil.

A Simple Eating Technique That Restores Enzymes and Fiber to Cooked Foods

You can overcome some of the drawbacks of cooked foods by eating a large salad of raw vegetables immediately before consuming a cooked course. This gives you plenty of fiber and enzymes to work through your digestive tract ahead of the cooked course. Make sure the salad is substantial. Eat it all before starting on the cooked course. And finish the cooked course only if you are still hungry.

Len R. Overcomes Arthritis While Continuing to Eat the Cooked Foods He Loves

Len R. was a stocky former football player who loved "good food." By his mid-fifties, Len's love had added 60 surplus pounds to his already heavy frame, and he began to experience pain in his hips, knees, and spine. His doctor said he had osteoarthritis and advised him to lose weight.

Len went right on eating the cooked foods he loved. But his wife Celeste, who came from Switzerland, had other ideas. She re-read some old German treatises on nature cure that had belonged to her father. The books described a subtle way to prepare food for people who refuse to change their diet.

Celeste began making soups, stews, baked dishes, and casseroles that tasted delicious but were low in fat. She preceded each meal with a raw vegetable salad. Len grumbled at the change in diet but admitted that the meals tasted good.

One morning, Len noticed that his pants seemed several inches too large around the waist. Lately, he'd also been feeling better. The pain in his joints had diminished, and he no longer needed laxatives.

Bit by bit, Celeste's salads grew larger and Len shed as much as three pounds per week. In a few months time his weight was back to normal and his arthritis pains had almost gone.

When Celeste explained it was all due to the change in diet, Len was finally convinced. He still continued to enjoy cooked foods. But by always eating a large salad first, Len transferred the benefits of living foods to the cooked foods he still loved.

Overcoming Arthritis the 65-20-15 Way

The 65-20-15 diet is recommended by most natural health practitioners as a way to maintain optimum health and heal arthritis.

Essentially, the 65-20-15 formula means that 65 percent of your calories are derived from complex carbohydrates, a maximum of 20 percent from fats, and 15 percent or so from protein. These ratios vary, of course, depending on your need and the seasons.

What the 65-20-15 formula does is to ensure a diet low in fat and high in fiber with an adequate supply of protein and an abundance of natural vitamins, minerals, and enzymes.

To give you a better idea of how much of each food type you should eat, follow this general guideline. Remember eat more fruits and vegetables in the summer and spring, and more of other foods during cold seasons. Percent of total volume also depends on climate, activity, and your individual needs.

Vegetables:	30 to 50 percent
Fruits:	10 to 25 percent
Grains, legumes, and beans:	20 to 40 percent
Animal products:	7 to 12 percent
Seeds and nuts:	5 to 8 percent

Although nothing in this book urges you to go vegetarian, should you decide to do so, increase the amount of protein-containing vegetarian foods proportionately.

Proteins That Restore Youthful Health

Protein should comprise 15 percent of your dietary calories. The one best sourse of whole protein for anyone with arthritis is cold-water fish such as haddock or salmon. Freshwater fish like mountain trout is also good if taken from unpolluted waters. Fattier fish contain natural inflammation fighting EPA. Buy fresh fish if you can: the flesh should be firm, the eyes bright, the scales shiny and there should be a strong, fresh, briny smell. Frozen fish is next best. Smoked fish should be strictly avoided. Many shellfish are high in saturated fat and should be eaten only occasionally.

Once frozen fish is thawed, it must be eaten immediately. If you freeze your own fish, wrap it in moisture vapor wrapping or glazing to prevent dehydration.

Cook fish over a low, gentle heat. Fish can be baked, broiled, sautéed, or poached and made into a casserole. Almost all fish are rich in B-complex and other vitamins and in calcium, copper, iodine, iron, magnesium, and phosphorous. Eat the bones if they are soft enough.

Good low-fat sources of whole protein are chicken and turkey without the skin (the white flesh is best); lean beef, veal and other very lean meats; and non-fat dairy foods like plain non-fat yogurt and cottage cheese. Baker's, Farmer's, and Hoop cheeses are also low in fat and cholesterol. Egg whites are another low-fat source of whole protein.

Although these foods are all low in fat and cholesterol, none contain any fiber or appreciable enzymes.

Proteins Without Cholesterol

If you are willing to take a little trouble, vegetarian protein is superior in many ways. All vegetable protein is cholesterol free, high in fiber, rich in enzymes and has an abundance of vitamins and minerals.

Good sources of vegetable protein are beans (especially soybeans), nuts (especially pecans), nuts, seeds, sprouts, and grains.

No vegetable food contains all eight essential amino acids which the body needs to synthesize whole protein. To get all eight, you must eat a variety of protein-containing plant foods within a day—not a difficult task if you're consuming a variety of foods.

With all its advantages, there are people who don't thrive on vegetable protein alone. If you're one who requires an occasional dose of low-fat, organic animal protein, help yourself. Let your body tell you how to eat.

Fresh Garden Vegetables Without Soil

Sprouts are seldom if ever allergenic and are rich in protein, vitamins, minerals, enzymes, and chlorophyll.

Chlorophyll is the living green color in all leafy, green vegetables which transforms sunlight into energy. Chlorophyll can literally be called a miracle food. A study at the University of Texas Systems Cancer Center in Houston identified chlorophyll as having powerful anti-cancer properties and it is a key nutrient in restoring health.

Almost all seeds, grains, and beans can be sprouted. Alfalfa and mung beans, available at all health food stores, are easiest to begin with.

Simply place a half-inch depth of seeds in the bottom of a wide-mouth jar and soak in water overnight. Cover the mouth with cheesecloth or screen. Then rinse and drain 2–3 times a day. In 3–5 days, the jar will be filled with fresh, crunchy sprouts. Wheat and large seeds may take 7–10 days to grow. Eat wheat sprouts while they are about an inch long, otherwise they acquire a strong taste.

Most sprouts grow best in a warm room in indirect sunlight. To turn them a rich green color, place them in full sunlight for the final day. This ensures they are rich in chlorophyll. Then store them in the refrigerator. Through sprouting, the original nutrient content of the seed is doubled or tripled. Sprouts are delicious in salads or sandwiches. They can also be lightly cooked.

Besides alfalfa and mung beans, you can sprout sunflower, pumpkin, squash, mustard, lettuce, peas, sesame, wheat, and many other seeds. Many health food stores carry inexpensive sprouting kits.

The Safe Way to Eat Fat

Our diets already contain too much fat for good health, hence the 65-20-15 formula seeks to restrict fat intake. Fat from seeds, nuts, whole grains, and avocados are free of cholesterol and low in rancidity.

High quality monounsaturated fat can also be obtained from cold-pressed, unrefined canola or stronger tasting olive oils. If you must fry foods, use one of these oils. Just be careful not to let the oil smoke—this creates harmful free radicals. Freshly squeezed, unsalted nuts are a good food provided they are eaten in moderation.

Safflower oil mayonnaise sold in health food stores is considered a reasonably safe source of fat. And, of course, don't forget your regular meals of fatty fish.

Shiela W.'s Arthritis Vanishes After Wonder Foods Sweep Out Her System

When Shiela W. was diagnosed as having rheumatoid arthritis, she was told to take 12 aspirins a day, to give up all exercise, and to rest.

Instead, Shiela consulted a clinical ecologist—an allergist who specializes in foods. The ecologist put Shiela on a 5-day fast and found she was allergic to chicken, potatoes, and cottage cheese. At both breakfast and dinner, she would feast on baked chicken with baked potatoes smothered in cottage cheese.

Although Shiela firmly believed in nutritional therapy, she could not bring herself to give up the baked chicken, potatoes, and cottage cheese. The ecologist tested Shiela's bowel transit time and found it took four days for these mainly low-fiber foods to pass through her gastrointestinal system. The ecologist realized immediately that partly digested particles of Shiela's allergic foods were passing into her bloodstream during their long, slow trip through her leaky intestines.

Shiela was advised to eat a large, raw fruit salad before her regular breakfast and an equally large raw vegetable salad before her regular dinner. She was also to eat three thick slices of whole grain bread with her chicken at both breakfast and dinner. Another test a week later showed that Shiela's bowel trip time had been reduced to only 30 hours.

As the ecologist had guessed, the bulk and fiber in the raw salads and bread swept boldly through Shiela's intestines carrying the low-residue cooked chicken, and cottage cheese, as well as potatoes along with it.

As the time these partially digested food particles spent in her intestines was cut, absorption of these foods into Shiela's bloodstream was also drastically reduced. This, in turn, cut the allergic reaction by Shiela's immune system and it eased the autoimmune attack on her joints.

Eventually, Shiela was able to drop the allergic foods altogether and to replace them with nuts, seeds, and avocados. In the three years since she took this step, she has stayed completely free of arthritis symptoms.

Complex Carbohydrates— Nature's Miracle Anti-Arthritis Food

Sixty to eighty percent of all restorative foods should consist of fresh, living fruits, vegetables, and whole grains. Because large amounts of fruit sugar can temporarily unbalance blood sugar levels, most nutritionists recommend eating at least twice as many vegetables and grains as fruits.

Fruits, and particularly citrus, are good sources of vitamin C, often called the arthritis vitamin because of its widespread role in arthritis recovery. Deep colored berries and cherries are also healing. So you need at least four fruits or fruit selections per day. Other fruits considered beneficial in arthritis recovery are bananas, apricots, and melons.

Try to avoid eating the skins of fruits that have been sprayed with pesticide. However, the skins of apples and similar fruits have such nutritional value that they should be eaten if at all possible. You can remove some of the pesticide residue by scrubbing fruit skins with a wire brush or buy organic produce.

Also peel the skins of vegetables like cucumbers that may have been sprayed and then rubbed with oil by supermarket personnel. You can remove most of the pesticide residue from lettuce, celery, and similar vegetables by removing the outer leaves or stalks and cutting off the top. This expedient is regrettable because many of the nutrients are contained in the skin. Again, patronize stores that carry organic foods.

Another solution is to start your own organic garden and grow your own produce.

Free Radicals Ignite Arthritis

Arthritis, and other degenerative diseases, are also being blamed on free radicals, highly reactive molecules produced by your body and the environment. It's the free radical's unpaired electron that makes trouble, as it scrounges for a partner—almost any molecule will do—before it will rest. This snatching up of protein and other bystanders by free radicals damage cells and tissues, is the basis for arthritic aches and aging.

The first and largest source of free radicals is your own body, odd considering the harm they cause. Your body uses oxygen to burn food and create energy, not unlike blowing on a smoldering fire to increase its flame. Free radicals are the sparks that fly off this metabolic blaze. Your body stomps out free radical sparks with its own stockpile of firefighters called antioxidants including glutathione and superoxide dismutase.

However, free radicals are exceedingly helpful in the right amounts. In a sense, they're part of your immune system. White blood cells harness free radicals to disarm invading germs, and the liver uses them for detoxifying hurtful toxins. It's ironic then that an aging, faltering immune system is partly due to free radical overload[50].

In today's world it's easy to push your burden of free radicals over the top with pollution, too much sun, pesticides, radiation, some drugs, cigarettes, and stressor foods like alcohol and rancid fats. These stresses also eat up antioxidants and other nutrients. When free radicals climb too high or antioxidants fall too low, chronic diseases like arthritis are more likely to ignite. Richard Cutler, PhD, investigator at the Gerontology Research Center of the National Institute on Aging, says studies suggest an almost linear relationship between lifespan and antioxidant levels in some animals[51].

Antioxidant-Containing Foods to the Rescue

Luckily Mother Nature has handed us a shopping cart of full restorative-antioxidant foods that disarm free radicals. Over 4000 free radical-fighting plant pigments called flavonoids have been identified[52]. Yellow, red, and darker colored vegetables get their pigment partially from carotene, some of nature's best known antioxidants. Paler vegetables like iceberg lettuce don't pack nearly the punch that dark leafy greens do.

Among food families, cruciferous vegetables are considered valuable in arthritis nutrition because they contain indoles, another substance believed to have antioxidant power. Broccoli, cauliflower, Brussels sprouts, and their cruciferous cousins seldom cause allergies.

The carotene called lycopene is high in tomatoes. Leeks, kiwi, and spinach are good reservoirs of another coloring carotene, lutein. More than 500 carotenes have been catalogued to date.

Most vegetables quickly lose their nutrients when they wilt. So pack them in plastic bags to keep them fresh longer. Try sticking to fresh vegetables; frozen are second best.

Whole, fresh fruit provides another warehouse of wonder nutrients. Terpenes are the antioxidants found in citrus fruits, like grapefruit and limes. Brightly colored fruits like oranges and papaya hold both flavonoids and carotenes.

Don't forget to eat legumes including beans, peas, soybeans, and lentils. Besides being valuable protein foods, the isoflavones and lectins in these delectable dishes provide antioxidant protection against arthritis-provoking free radicals.

Health-Promoting Properties of Other Common Foods

Whole grains are an excellent source of fiber and B-vitamins. Coarsely cut oatmeal is a recommended breakfast cereal and takes only a few minutes to cook in a double boiler. Serve with fruit or raisins; add a few nuts or seeds, or a dollop of non-fat yogurt.

Most commercially packaged cereals have a high sugar content, including granola (which is also high in fat). Several brands are sugar-free, and health food and grocery stores carry healthier versions of many popular breakfast cereals.

Bread made exclusively of whole grain flour minus the additives and sugar is a good health-restoring food. Yeast-free breads like unleavened bread and pita bread or chapatis are less likely to be allergenic.

Follow the 3-S rule and eat several, small, simple meals each day. For snacks, chew on carrots, radishes, jicama, or other raw crunchy vegetables. Try sunflower seeds and nuts mixed with dried fruit. Apples, pears, or other succulent fruit alone or mixed with yogurt is very satisfying.

All these wholesome foods are delicious and will keep your mouth happy and your body healthy. Such restorative foods are jammed with vitamins and minerals including antioxidant vitamins C and E, and selenium.

The 65-20-15 Formula Galvanizes Jane R.'s Body into Throwing Off Arthritis

Jane R. was 45 when she was divorced. Soon afterwards, osteoarthritis appeared in the joints of her fingers and toes. Pea-shaped knobs began to form on the end joints of her fingers, and her doctor diagnosed them as Heberden's nodes. On each hand, the tips of her index and small fingers began to turn in towards the middle finger.

Her doctor's prognosis that nothing could be done sent Jane inquiring about alternative therapies. A friend who had had both hypertension and gout told Jane that, after changing his diet to over-come hypertension, the gout had also disappeared. The diet was the 65-20-15 formula which is often used by nutritionists in treating high blood pressure.

Under her friend's guidance, Jane changed over to a diet in which 85 percent of her food consisted of fruits, vegetables, legumes, beans, and grains; 5 percent of nuts, seeds, and avocados; and 10 percent of fish and chicken. (These food amounts are approximate, but did fulfill the 65-20-15 guidelines.)

Within a week, the 65-20-15 formula abruptly ended several minor ailments that had plagued Jane for years. Her chronic irregularity was replaced by easy, thrice-daily bowel movements. She no longer had frequent headaches. And her heartburn and acid stomach quickly disappeared.

Jane was so encouraged by these results that she stuck right with the 65-20-15 formula. Her roly-poly body gradually began to firm up, and in eight weeks her figure was slim and trim.

At this point, she noticed that the pain and stiffness in her fingers and toes had disappeared. The disfiguring bony protuberances remained. But normal use of her fingers and toes had been completely restored.

Today, 5 years later, Jane continues to eat the 65-20-15 way. Her overall health has improved tremendously. She now plays tennis regularly and swims a mile nonstop three times each week. The only reminders of her bout with arthritis are the flat, spatulated joints at the ends of her fingers and toes.

Unusual Benefits from Unusual Beverages

For beverages, try some freshly-squeezed vegetable juices. They are preferable to fruit juices. Carrot juice goes particularly well with breakfast. You can juice vegetables in a juicer or blender. Carbonated spring water mixed with a little fruit juice is a good substitute for soft drinks.

For a hot beverage, try carob or herbal teas. Carob is a chocolate-like drink. Make sure the brand you buy is sugar-free.

The following teas are beneficial for arthritis: alfalfa, boneset, chamomile, celery, linden, parsley, peppermint, and wintergreen leaves. You can sweeten any hot drink with a little honey. (See Chapter 14 for more ideas.)

Particularly recommended is chamomile tea as a natural relaxant and sedative. It induces drowsiness and sleep and helps people with arthritis get a good night's sleep. It also helps digestion.

If your drinking water is heavily treated, or has tested allergy-positive, drink only bottled or filtered water.

Try to rotate all foods so they are eaten about four days apart. For example, you might eat walnuts one day, almonds the second day, Brazils the third day, and cashews the fourth day. It is not always possible to space out foods this far apart. But at least try to avoid eating a lot of any one food frequently. They *could* become allergenic if you are predisposed to allergies.

Eat Only Compatible Foods

Naturally, you should omit from your list of restorative foods any that you have tested out as allergy-positive. After an abstinence of several weeks along with a rehabilitated digestive tract, you may be able to eat some of them again at well-spaced-out intervals.

If you are living or eating with a family or group who continue to eat stressor foods, you must separate your food from theirs. You need your own part of the refrigerator for fresh fruits and vegetables and you may find a pressure cooker useful.

Easing Smoothly into Living Foods

Suppose you have another ailment which is aggravated by uncooked foods. In reality, very few ailments, including ulcers and gall bladder problems, are really irritated by uncooked foods. However, for some conditions like ulcerative colitis and Crohn's disease it is dangerous to eat high fiber, raw, rough foods during a flare-up. Check with your doctor.

If you do experience any digestive problems, make a gradual transition from your present low-bulk, all-cooked diet to high-fiber restorative foods. Make the changeover gradually and in easy stages. Many people with digestive problems find it takes about six weeks to make the changeover. By that time, all their digestive problems have usually disappeared.

Naturally, if you are under medical care or taking medication for any ailment that might be affected by a change in diet, you should consult your doctor first.

Stay at the Peak of Good Health the Rest of Your Life

Be prepared to stay with restorative foods permanently. With a cyclical allergy you can cheat occasionally and get away with it. Repairing your GI tract often solves many food intolerances too. But people who stray back to fixed allergy foods often experience a flare-up of arthritis symptoms the following morning.

Whenever our health is at its highest peak, our resistance to arthritis is greatest. Fit, healthy people succumb to arthritis less often. An arthritis sufferer who attains the peak of health is able to shake off arthritis sooner or at the very least, reduce pain.

Thus the obvious way to prevent or to reverse arthritis is to live at the peak of good health all of the time.

The Dozen Health-Renewing Powers of Restorative Foods

Most professional healers in charge of arthritis clinics today consider that the disease is the result of nutritional deficiencies.

For example, Robert Bingham, M.D., medical director of the National Arthritis Medical Clinic at Desert Hot Springs, California, states: "It has been found that seven out of ten patients with arthritis will improve or recover after changes in their dietary habits. The type and quality of food intake of a patient with arthritis is extremely important. Most patients with arthritis have unrecognized dietary deficiencies and personal nutrition problems. Some patients lack essential items in their diet especially natural proteins, vitamins, minerals, and enzymes. Some patients are underweight because of poor appetite, pain, and the use of drugs. Others are overweight from consuming an excess of sugars and fats or from an inability to exercise because of joint pain and stiffness."

Osteoarthritis, for instance, occurs when the bones, tissue, and cartilage in a joint are weakened by nutritional deficiencies. At the same time, a nutritionally poor diet may cause the victim to become overweight. When this excess weight is superimposed on the nutritionally weakened joint, the resulting wear and tear breaks down the bone, tissue, and cartilage, creating the condition known as osteoarthritis.

Osteoarthritis can be improved only by changing to a diet of nutritionally-rich restorative foods. By restoring sound nutrition, the victim's weight gradually drops back to normal while the joint is also gradually able to restore itself from the abundant supply of essential nutrients available in the bloodstream.

How do restorative foods make good the various dietary deficiencies and other dysfunctions brought about by arthritis?

#1. By Restoring the Vitamin-Mineral-Enzyme Deficiency That Afflicts Almost Everyone with Arthritic Disease

Almost all men and women with any degree of severe arthritis have a serious deficiency of B-complex vitamins; vitamins A, C, D, and E; and the minerals calcium, magnesium, manganese, and zinc. Studies show that B-vitamin blood levels in persons with arthritis are as much as 75 percent lower than in the general population. This routine deficiency deprives the body of many nutrients needed to keep the cells of joints, tissue, bone, and muscle healthy.

For example, a deficiency of minerals like calcium, magnesium, manganese, and zinc restricts production of synovial fluid, inhibiting lubrication in arthritic joints.

Deficiencies of vitamin C and calcium have such serious effects that they must be considered separately.

Not only arthritis patients but almost all Americans 50 and over suffer from some degree of vitamin, mineral, and enzyme deficiency. It is well established that stomach acid, required for some nutrient breakdown and absorption, declines with age[53]. Also, fat laden animal foods nowadays contain significantly fewer nutrients than they did several decades ago when animals were leaner and healthier. Yet basic nutrition handbooks published by the government continue to quote vitamin and mineral contents of animal foods based on research done decades ago.

For example, it was recently found that modern pork contains 30 percent less iron than formerly, while modern beef has 20 percent less. Today's animals are simply fatter than in earlier times and the more fat in an animal, the fewer nutrients its meaty tissues contain.

Again, refined foods are often enriched with supplements that are less biologically usable by the body than natural nutrients. Also these foods that are enriched, like refined flour and whole-fat milk, are often high-risk stressor foods and should not be eaten anyway.

Restorative Foods are Rich in Health-Building Nutrients

While millions of people do take vitamin and mineral supplements, they are second choice to nutrient-rich foods. Before supplements can be utilized by the body, for instance, most mineral supplements must be adequately formed with complexes of amino acid or protein chelates. Single B vitamins like B_6 are most beneficial when taken together with all other B-complex vitamins. And B_6 cannot be utilized unless zinc is present. Too much of one nutrient can actually throw another off balance. For example, long-term, high doses of zinc may upset copper levels.

Calcium cannot be utilized unless adequate amounts of vitamin D are present. Nor can calcium be utilized well when the body's phosphorous level is too high. Many stressor foods like carbonated drinks have high levels of phosphorus and low levels of calcium. As a result, arthritis patients who eat large amounts of animal protein or drink a lot of soda often have such low calcium levels that after several years, they lose their teeth and show a serious loss of skeletal bone.

The requirements for proper absorption of vitamin and mineral supplements are often so exacting that most people are better off obtaining their vitamins and minerals from natural foods. Provided the foods are low in fat and high in fiber, the mix of vitamins and minerals is so varied that the right proportion of most nutrients is readily available. The old adage of "the more you know, the more you realize you don't know" applies perfectly to nutrition. Scientists are discovering new food nutrients every year. Meaning, if you only rely on pills for your vitamins, minerals, and fiber you're guaranteed to be missing something. (Having said this, realize too that there is a place for vitamin pills in arthritis treatment.)

Absorption difficulties and digestive problems occur less frequently with restorative foods. In fruits, vegetables, nuts, seeds, and grains, all minerals are naturally chelated, with better absorption almost assured. And all of these living foods are rich in enzymes helpful for digestion.

Dottie L. Discovers Amazing Benefits from Calcium-Rich Restorative Foods

"I was a heavy eater of sugar, white bread, pastries, and junk food." This is 45-year-old Dottie L. speaking. "By my fortieth birthday, I had pain and stiffness in my left knee, my neck, and the wrists and fingers of both hands. Eventually I could hardly walk. My doctor diagnosed it as rheumatoid arthritis.

"The doctor told me to replace the refined foods with lots of meat, chicken, and eggs and to cut out all dairy foods. This helped some. But my joints just became stiffer and nodules began to appear.

"It was obvious I wasn't getting any better. So I went to see a chiropractor who specializes in nutrition. He had me fast for five days, and I tested allergic to chicken, wheat, beef, and yeast." She was also told her diet lacked certain minerals like magnesium and zinc.

"I was advised to drop all high-protein foods and to eat mainly fresh fruits, grains, and produce. The chiropractor said to eat plenty of low-fat yogurt and cruciferous vegetables to build up my calcium. I also took vitamin D."

"Well, only 15 days after the fast, and my joint pains had almost disappeared. A month later I could walk and use my arms and wrists freely."

Gradually, the worst of the nodules disappeared. Now, three years later, Dottie still has some disfigurement. But she remains free of pain as long as she stays with her diet, and she is more active than she has been since her teens.

#2. By Restoring Collagen Integrity

Arthritis has long been linked with collagen abnormality. Collagen, a body protein, comprises two thirds of all cartilage in our joints and it plays a vital role in the health of each joint and its supportive tissues.

The marginal nutrition supplied by stressor foods reduces the total amount of collagen in the connective tissues of each joint. Collagen breakdown is made worse by insufficient of vitamins A, B_6, and C and the minerals magnesium and zinc. Vitamin C is absolutely essential in the formation and maintenance of collagen. Vitamin B_6, also essential for collagen production, must be eaten daily together with other B-complex vitamins.

All of these nutrients are supplied in abundance by such restorative foods as fresh fruits, vegetables, nuts, seeds, and whole grains.

#3. By *Improving Calcium Utilization*

Many people with arthritic disease have a severe calcium deficiency. Whenever calcium levels in food and in the bloodstream are low, a hormone from the parathyroid gland called parathormone triggers release of calcium from skeletal bones. Too much of this over the years contributes to excessive bone loss known as osteoporosis.

The calcium which is leached from bones and teeth may deposit in arthritic joints. This leaves the bones demineralized, fragile, brittle, and easily broken. Osteoporosis is most common among middle-aged and older postmenopausal women—some with arthritis. Chinese researchers from the Shantou University Medical School found that 30 percent of their older arthritic patients were also afflicted with osteoporosis[54].

Osteoporosis can be hastened by eating more animal protein than the body can handle. Studies have shown that women who eat large amounts of meat, eggs, and poultry lose 35 percent of their skeletal bone mass between ages 50 and 89, while vegetarian women lose only 18 percent. These tests show that a high protein diet may double bone loss.

Nutritional studies have also proved that eating foods high in bone building nutrients like calcium and vitamin D, as well as magnesium, boron, and vitamins K, B_{12}, B_6 and folic acid, fend off osteoporosis. You might think bones are just sticks that hold the body up. The truth is, bones are living, changing tissues that need just as many vitamins and minerals as other organs. Too much protein, salt, alcohol, and caffeine[53] also harm bones.

The trick to keeping bones healthy is to start young—preferably before age 35. The earlier you stockpile bones with calcium and other nutrients, the stronger your skeleton will be later on. This doesn't mean, however, that you should abandon nutritious eating once you reach 40. Quite the contrary. A physically active life and restorative foods may not give you 30-year-old bones, but they will slow down or prevent further bone loss and perhaps help you regain a little of the bone you've already lost.

Take the 1991 study at Tufts University in Boston where post-menopausal women who walked regularly and upped their calcium intake for one year recovered a modest amount of bone[55].

Restorative foods are naturally rich in all bone nutrients. Green leafy vegetables are bursting with vitamin K, calcium, magnesium, and the B vitamins. Whole grains have more magnesium and B vitamins. Various nuts contain both calcium and magnesium. Fruits and vegetables hold plenty of boron, and soybeans and cauliflower are vitamin K reservoirs. Vitamin D, needed by your body to utilize calcium, can be obtained by sunbathing for about 15 minutes daily. Fatty fish, great pain and inflammation relievers, are also warehouses of vitamin D.

#4. By Restoring Vitamin C Deficiency

According to a report in *Annals of the Rheumatic Diseases* (Vol. 50, No. 2, 1991) a British research team found blood drawn from patients with rheumatoid arthritis was less proficient at protecting its cells from the ravages of free radical molecules when compared to healthy individuals. Vitamin C—a prominent antioxidant that disarms destructive free radicals—was also lower in the arthritis group[56].

Vitamin C, the chief custodian of collagen, is a powerful healer which is present in generous quantities in a healthy person's adrenal glands. But vitamin C is so lacking in people with arthritic disease that, in a study at the Department of Pharmacology at Trinity College, Dublin, Ireland, it was found that 85 percent of all people with rheumatoid arthritis were actually suffering from subclinical scurvy. The researchers found that vitamin C is consumed faster in people with arthritis than in healthy people. One reason is that aspirin leaches vitamin C from the blood. In doing so, it suppresses the immune system and lowers resistance to all infectious diseases. Free radical overload—typical in arthritis—also eats up vitamin C reserves.

Stressor foods are particularly deficient in vitamin C.

This lack of vitamin C is believed to be one factor causing the abnormality in the immune system that recognizes harmless food particles as foreign invaders. A deficiency of vitamin C also exacerbates joint problems while an abundance of vitamin C helps ease stress in joints.

By following the 65-20-15 formula, up to 65 percent of a restorative food diet consists of fresh fruits and vegetables with ample nutritive ability to restore the deficiency of vitamin C in the average arthritis patient.

#5. By Normalizing the Immune Response

Rheumatoid arthritis may occur when, through an abnormality, the white cells of the immune system identify food particles as foreign and then mistakenly attack the cells in your joints. This abnormality occurs less often in a totally healthy person with optimum nutrition.

Poor nutrition is a frequent cause of immune system suppression and abnormality. For example, research at such renowned institutions as Memorial Sloan-Kettering Cancer Center and the City of Hope National Medical Center in Duarte, California, have demonstrated that performance of the immune system can be bolstered by an abundant supply of vitamin C and zinc together with adequate amounts of vitamins A and E and the B-complex. Several research scientists have hypothesized that this nutritional boost will also help eliminate the abnormal reactions that lead to arthritis.

Restorative foods rich in vitamin C are leafy, green vegetables, citrus fruits, strawberries, broccoli, Brussels sprouts, tomatoes, turnip, cabbage, cantaloupe and honeydew melon, okra, potatoes, and sweet red peppers. Zinc, a trace element, is present in many vegetables and grains. Carrots are rich in vitamin A. And such foods as seeds, nuts, grains, and leafy, green vegetables are good sources of B-complex vitamins.

Jack F. Ends Excruciating Gout with Health-Promoting Foods

At age 55, Jack F. had suffered from increasingly severe episodes of gout for over ten years. On his doctor's advice, Jack stopped eating foods high in purines. His attacks did become less frequent. But every few weeks, the joints in his feet and ankles would suddenly become hot, swollen, tender, and throbbing, and the pain would last for several days.

Finally, a friend got Jack interested in nutrition. Although Jack had stopped eating foods high in purines, his diet still included large amounts of canned and cooked foods with almost no fresh fruits or produce. The friend advised Jack to cut out all foods that were refined, canned, and processed and to replace them with natural foods containing vitamin C. Jack was also advised to eat plenty of leafy, green vegetables, pecans, soybeans, and brown rice for their B-complex vitamins.

One full year after Jack changed his diet, he did not experience a single gout attack. When his doctor checked Jack's uric acid levels, they had dropped back to normal.

The explanation? Jack's nutritionist friend believes that vitamin C increases excretion of uric acid in the purine. But we must not forget, either, that Jack had also stopped eating most stressor foods and had replaced them with a diet of natural restorative foods. The chances are that, in doing so, he also removed the underlying cause of his gout.

#6. By Decreasing Free Radical Load and Loading Up on Antioxidant-Rich Foods

Free radicals are made by your body and used by white blood cells to kill germs; the liver employs them for detoxifying hurtful toxins. It's ironic then that these same free radical molecules—without which you'd die—can in high amounts make arthritis worse.

Unfortunately, chronic inflammation, in and of itself a sign that your immune system is hard at work, creates a mass of free radicals that overwhelm your body's antioxidant reserves.

One way to reduce free radical load is by avoiding situations and substances that produce these molecules. The other, says Bruce Ames, PhD, director of the National Institutes of Environmental Health Sciences Center at the University of California, Berkeley, is to feast on antioxidant-rich fruits and vegetables. People who eat at least five servings of produce daily versus those consuming few or none get cancer half as often, and have considerably fewer cataracts and heart problems[57].

#7. By Improving Elimination and Slowing Absorption of Toxins and Food Particles into the Bloodstream

No food of animal origin contains any fiber and all stressor foods are low-residue foods, meaning they pass slowly through the digestive system and are excreted as small, hard feces. Expelling these feces often causes straining and for some hemorrhoids. So it is hardly surprising to learn that many arthritis patients suffer from poor elimination.

In fact, stressor foods are so low in fiber (also called roughage or bulk) that they take 2–5 days to pass through the digestive system compared to slightly more than a day for restorative foods.

This long transit time in the intestines allows far more partially digested food particles to be absorbed into the bloodstream where they overload the liver, may set off the immune response, and spark arthritis in the susceptible.

Less fiber upsets microbial balance in the bowel. A long, slow transit time also gives pathogenic or disease-causing bacteria in the intestines more time to break down decayed fecal matter and turn it into toxins that are also absorbed into the bloodstream. When this happens, other body organs such as the skin, lungs, and kidneys are called on to eliminate the toxins. The breath becomes malodorous, perspiration smells offensive, the skin is dry and rough, and the urine becomes dark and smelly. These signs of poor elimination are common in people with arthritis.

Nature's Cleansing Broom

These facts were medically confirmed by British researcher Dr. Dennis Burkitt and his colleagues while studying the effects of dietary fiber on colon cancer. They theorized that a high fiber diet protects against colon cancer by shortening the time food wastes take to pass through the digestive system. They found that in Africans living on natural, high-fiber diets, stools are so large and move through the intestines so rapidly that hazardous toxins are diluted and waste matter is quickly eliminated.

By comparison, the hard, sluggish stools of people in western industrial nations who consume large amounts of stressor foods pass so slowly through the intestines that bacteria are able to break down the natural bile acids and turn them into carcinogens that cause colon cancer.

Writing in the *Journal of the American Medical Association* as far back as 1974, Dr. Burkitt stated his belief that lack of dietary fiber in refined foods and animal-derived foods is at least a partial cause of most degenerative diseases.

Conventional practitioners continue to debate about fiber's role in health. As they do, a mounting pile of studies confirm that diets low in roughage contribute to constipation, diabetes, obesity, Crohn's disease, gallstones, peptic ulcers, diverticular disease, and high cholesterol[58].

You can easily check your own transit time like this. After dinner, swallow some unchewed raw corn; or chew and swallow a whole cooked beet; or eat some blueberries. These markers will show up in the feces allowing you to check the exact length of transit time. The corn will appear exactly as you ate it; the beets will leave an unmistakable deep red color; and the blueberries will color the stool blue-green.

If your transit time is more than 36 hours, your diet is low in fiber. A diet of typical restorative foods will pass in 15–30 hours with large, soft, unimpacted stools that sweep toxins and waste matter clear out of the intestines.

Arthritis—The Cooked Food Disease

During a study in South Africa, it was found that while the bowel transit time for Europeans on a diet of low-residue foods averaged 90 hours, transit took only 18-24 hours for Africans on a raw diet of high-fiber foods. But when the Africans ate the same foods cooked, their transit time increased to 35 hours.

Cooking is another form of food processing that destroys many enzymes in foods; it breaks down some fiber in some foods; it destroys some vitamins entirely; and many other vitamins and minerals are lost in cooking water. Because it destroys some fiber, cooking is also one contribution to constipation—a condition common in people with arthritis.

Just how detrimental cooking is to health was demonstrated in a classic experiment in 1946 by Dr. Francis Pottenger, an M.D. on the faculty of the University of California at Berkeley. Dr. Pottenger divided several hundred cats into two groups. One group was exclusively fed cooked meats and pasteurized milk while the other group got raw meat and raw milk.

Pottenger found that the group on the cooked diet developed a variety of food allergies along with arthritis and other degenerative diseases. Their immune systems were also suppressed to where they became susceptible to a variety of infections including pneumonia.

Dr. Pottenger found that the cooked food cats soon acquired the same ailments as humans eating the western industrialized diet. They became listless and fatigued. Many showed signs of diabetes, and as time went on, arthritis became widespread.

Many cooked food cats died while giving birth and their offspring were sickly and weak. Each generation showed more food allergies than the last. By the fourth generation, the cooked food cats were no longer able to reproduce.

Meanwhile, the raw food cats enjoyed optimum health and thrived.

Dr. Edward Howell, of Illinois and Florida, a pioneer researcher in enzymes, also found that cooked food passes through the colon more slowly than raw food. During the extended transit time, cooked food ferments causing gas, bloating, headaches, and colon diseases. Many colon specialists estimate that the average middle-aged meat-eating American who consumes most foods cooked is carrying a 3-4 day build up of waste fecal matter on his or her intestinal walls that weighs from 8–30 pounds. This excess weight causes the colon to stretch and sag while toxic wastes seep into the bloodstream through leaky intestinal walls. During colonic irrigations, large quantities of hard, black fecal debris and cord-like mucous are expelled.

Chronic constipation can be permanently reversed in a few days to a couple of weeks by changing to a diet of restorative foods.

#8. By Normalizing Weight

The immediate cause of most cases of osteoarthritis is wear and tear on joints often caused by the burden of carrying surplus weight. When a changeover is made from a conventional diet of high-fat, low-fiber stressor foods to a low-fat, high-fiber diet of restorative foods, the total intake of calories is sharply reduced.

Studies of people who eat a high-fiber diet of restorative foods show that while such a diet is filling and satisfying, it is usually low in fat and calories. Indications are, also, that with an exclusively high-fiber diet, the body absorbs fewer calories from the digestive tract thus maintaining weight at an optimum level.

As restorative foods begin to rebalance body chemistry, one of the immediate results is to normalize the mechanisms that control appetite and weight through carbohydrate metabolism via the pancreas.

Recovering from osteoarthritis through weight loss is covered in detail in Chapter 15. Persons with rheumatoid or similar forms of arthritis who have lost weight find that restorative foods will gradually rebuild their weight to the optimum level.

Restorative Foods Overcome a Severe Case of Osteoarthritis of the Spine

At age 55, Sarah D. had had osteoarthritis of the spine for over five years. She was 30 pounds overweight. As a result of this excessive poundage, arthritis symptoms were already appearing in her knees.

What made it all worse was Sarah's chronic constipation. She rarely had a normal bowel movement. Once a week she would lie on the bathroom floor and give herself an enema. Afterwards, the toilet bowl was filled with hard, black fecal matter and stringy, cord-like excreta.

The explanation lay in Sarah's diet. She was inordinately fond of canned tuna fish, salmon, and sardines—not bad in and of themselves—but when served on toasted white bread with potato chips and mayonnaise, it made these meals less than wholesome. Eggs, cheese, hamburger, hot dogs, pies, pastries, ice cream, and coffee loomed large in the rest of her diet. She ate absolutely no fruits, vegetables, nuts, seeds, or whole grains, and her intake of fiber was near zero.

In the end, Sarah acquired the worst case of grapevine hemorrhoids her doctor had seen. Her stools were bloody and after each bowel movement, she had to push the hemorrhoids back inside her anus with her fingers.

Her sister had long been advising Sarah to change to a diet of natural foods. Sarah was so shaken by the hemorrhoids that she finally decided to take the plunge.

What her sister essentially advised was to give up all of the high-fat, low-fiber foods that are also often stressor foods and to replace them with a low-fat, high-fiber diet identical with our restorative foods.

Results were dramatic! Sarah's constipation, which had plagued her for half a lifetime, ended abruptly in just 48 hours. In place of the low-residue canned and refined foods that had taken a week to complete a bowel transit, the fiber-rich fruits, vegetables, grains, nuts, and seeds she now ate swept lustily through her digestive system in a bare 24 hours.

Sarah no longer had to strain at stools. She went to the bathroom regularly every eight hours. Her stools were bulky, soft, and totally unimpacted.

Most astounding was the effect on Sarah herself. She felt better than she had in years. Without dieting or watching calories, her weight fell by two pounds each week and her spine and knees began to improve.

In four months, her weight was back to normal and her arthritis symptoms were fast disappearing. The hemorrhoids seemed better too.

Complete recovery took a full year. By that time, Sarah was able to walk several miles without pain or fatigue. She could bend her spine easily in all directions. And her hemorrhoids were no longer a problem.

#9. *Through Boosting Production of Natural Cortisone by the Adrenal Glands*

Many forms of arthritis are helped by increasing output of the hormone cortisone from the adrenal glands. Medical science capitalizes on this by injecting cortisone derivatives in the form of corticosteroids (steroids) into joint tissue to suppress arthritic inflammation and pain or giving steroid pills. But when introduced artificially, cortisone throws the body out of balance, creating destructive and often life-threatening side effects.

Without going too deeply into the body chemistry involved, it has been found that foods rich in B-complex vitamins and vitamin C can naturally stimulate the adrenal glands into releasing large amounts of cortisone.

Dr. C. E. Barton-Wright, a well known rheumatologist, has speculated that both osteo and rheumatoid arthritis are basically the result of a deficiency of vitamins B_2 and B_6. These vitamins, together with vitamin C, stimulate the pituitary gland to release the hormone ACTH which triggers the release of increased amounts of natural cortisone by the adrenals.

The cortisone hormones released by the adrenals diminish inflammation and destruction of cartilage in joints without any of the side effects of artificial hormones.

Restorative foods like fruits, vegetables, nuts, seeds, and grains contain ample supplies of vitamin C and the B-complex vitamins that increase the output of adrenal cortisone.

#10. By Restoring Normal Blood Circulation to Arthritic Joints

Atherosclerosis, or hardening of the arteries, is egged on by a diet high in saturated fats and hydrogenated vegetable oils. Eating these stressful foods throws the body off balance, leading to deposits of LDL cholesterol in arteries throughout the body. As these fatty deposits clog arteries and restrict the flow of blood, oxygen, and essential nutrients to joints, the joints eventually weaken.

Cardiac rehabilitation programs have proved that atherosclerosis can be reversed by a low-fat diet high in fiber-rich complex carbohydrates. These restorative foods cleanse out the arteries and bring more blood and nutrients to inflamed joints and tissue.

#11. By Decreasing Inflammation Naturally

Saponin, a natural steroid-like compound found in many medicinal and eatable plants, has a direct anti-inflammatory effect on joints afflicted with rheumatoid arthritis. Although saponins vary greatly in action and chemical composition, most are not, or are hardly, absorbed across an intact gastrointestinal wall[59]. Some doctors speculate that saponins, perhaps related to this property, also reduce absorption of partly digested food particles and bacterial toxins into the bloodstream, thereby reducing autoimmune attack on joints.

It's the saponins in plants, like wild yam and soybeans, that provide drug companies with raw materials to manufacture cortisone—a powerful anti-inflammatory arthritis medicine—and other synthetic hormones[60]. Whether our bodies can convert basic plant steroids into human-like hormones is unknown. But the possibility exists.

The benefits of saponin were first revealed in a study reported in the *Journal of Applied Nutrition* (Vol. 27, No. 2 and 3, 1975) by rheumatologist Dr. Robert Bingham (an orthopedic surgeon and Medical Director of the National Arthritis Medical Center at Desert Hot

Springs, California) and Dr. Bernard Bellew (physician and operator of an arthritic clinic in Desert Hot Springs, California). In the double-blind Bingham-Bellew study, 165 arthritis patients, ranging in age from 11 to 92, received supplements containing saponin and other nutrients obtained from a local desert plant or else they were given placebos.

Little effect was noted by those who received placebos, but 60.7 percent of those receiving the saponin supplements reported significant relief of pain, swelling, and stiffness. Drs. Bingham and Bellew concluded: "In both osteo and rheumatoid forms of arthritis, (saponin) proved to have overall and specific beneficial effects."

In a similar study reportedly carried out by Dr. Robert A. Elliot of Woodland Hills, California, 50 percent of patients reported noticeable relief after taking saponin-containing supplements. Another rheumatologist, Dr. Paul Isaacson of Tucson, Arizona, is also reported to have found that 50–90 percent of his patients found some relief after taking saponin-containing tablets.

None of these doctors used saponin supplements alone. But all agreed that the saponin-containing supplements increased the success of other types of treatment also.

Since that first exciting study over 20 years ago, saponins, along with other phytochemicals have drawn the attention of many researchers. Nowadays saponins isolated from soybeans, ginseng, licorice, and other plants are demonstrating their potential for treating cancer[61], irregular heart beats[62], and atherosclerosis[63].

Perhaps the most relevant finding in relationship to arthritis is the healing effect various saponins have on the liver. Scientists from the University of Kansas discovered that saponins protect the liver from damage caused by acetaminophen (Tylenol™) overdose[64].

Saponin has been found to lower blood pressure, cholesterol, and blood fat levels. It also appears to reduce frequency of migraine and asthma attacks.

The most abundant source of saponin in the diet is soybeans. For instructions on how to use it, see "Recovery Food #7" in Chapter 14.

#12. By Enhancing the Growth of Friendly, Non-Toxic Bacteria

One way to crowd out toxic micro-organisms in your digestive tract is by enhancing the growth of friendly non-toxic bacteria.

Maintaining balance among the over 400 microbial species housed in your gut is vital for intestinal health.

Replacing these toxin-producing intestinal bacteria with beneficial ones reduces toxicity in the liver, bloodstream, and ultimately the joints.

The most natural way to realign gastrointestinal populations is by eating yogurt—a fermented milk product swimming with good bacteria. When a German research team, headed by Hans-Peter Bartram at the University of Wuerzburg, fed a dozen healthy individuals two cups of yogurt daily for three weeks, friendly bifidobacteria living in the GI tract increased significantly. An imbalance in intestinal bacteria, reported Bartram in a 1994 issue of the *American Journal of Clinical Nutrition* (Vol. 59), may enhance your risk of colon cancer[65].

All around the globe, scientists are celebrating the virtues of yogurt. In Italy, yogurt was found to increase intestinal production of IgA[66]—the same immunity factor lacking in many people with leaky gut syndrome. Children with persistent diarrhea, state Pakistan investigators, benefit from a yogurt diet[67].

And in this country at St. Joseph Health Center in St. Charles, Missouri, Marsha Johnson Schulte, a nurse specializing in cancer treatment, proclaimed that plain yogurt smeared on a smelly, ulcerated cancer sore for 10 minutes daily (along with antibiotic treatment) helped one of her patients. She exclaimed this natural treatment to be "cost-effective and . . . a rewarding experience for the patient and nursing staff"[68].

See Chapter 14, "Recovery Food" #14 for more information on this.

Chapter *14*

21 Wonderful Arthritis-Recovery Foods for the 21st Century

When interviewed years ago for a national periodical, Dr. Robert Bingham, Medical Director of the National Arthritis Medical Clinic in Desert Hot Springs, California, stated that a person with arthritis can significantly reduce pain and relieve stiffness and soreness in joints simply by eating foods containing essential vitamins, minerals, and enzymes.

The vitamins and minerals known to reduce pain include vitamins A, B-complex, C, D, and E and the minerals calcium and magnesium.

Dr. Bingham's findings are continually being confirmed by modern science. Researchers are re-discovering the curative powers of plants and herbs. Drug companies have confirmed that herbs like nettles are rich sources of vitamins, minerals, and healing enzymes while others like yucca and alfalfa contain steroid-like compounds.

As the yearly bill for health care hovers near $1,000, 000,000,000 dollars, government, employers and the general public are considering how foods and other therapies can enhance health. Once (and still) branded as quackery by many, the medicinal powers of food were given a stamp of approval in 1989 when the National Cancer Institute's Division of Cancer Prevention Control launched its five year $20.5 million dollar Experimental Foods Program, also known as the "Designer Foods" project. Arthritis-battling garlic, soybeans, and flaxseeds were just some of the foods studied.

Kristen McNutt, PhD, JD, a nutritional consultant from Ypsilanti, Michigan, puts it most aptly when she writes: "History will write that, approximately now, nutrition moved into a multi-decade era during which scientists eventually learned new ways of extending the quantity and enhancing the quality of life with food"[69].

Each of the 21 recovery foods described in this chapter has a special biochemical action that directly or indirectly affect joints. All are believed important in restoring the health of joint tissue, and all work naturally to help reverse arthritis.

Notwithstanding their undeniable therapeutic benefits, you can find these commonplace foods on the shelves of almost every supermarket or health food store.

Eat them as snacks or as part of your meals. But because these foods act as a tonic doesn't necessarily mean that the more you eat, the greater the effect. Take them in moderate amounts. And eat only when hungry.

For these foods to work naturally to help reverse arthritis, the cause must be removed first. So all stressor and allergy foods must be cut out in addition to using these foods before health is restored.

If you know or suspect that you have one or more of the dozen arthritis-linked nutrient deficiencies described in Chapter 13, by all means select one or more foods that you believe would help restore levels to normal. Then make them a regular part of your diet.

Naturally, you would not use any recovery foods to which you have tested allergy-positive. If you have any doubts as to whether you may have a sensitivity to any specific food, use the quick pulse test (Chapter 9) to find out.

Although we don't recommend eating any food too often, most recovery foods are so nutritionally beneficial that they can be eaten daily during recovery from arthritic disease. After that, you might use all of them less frequently on a rotating basis.

Recovery Food #1: Scientists Reveal the Anti-inflammatory and Immune Modulating Effects of Fish

For centuries fish-eating peoples have reaped the benefits of their marine diets. While typical American fare averages only 20 grams of fish a day, the Japanese thrive on five times that while native Greenland meals contain four times more than those in Japan[70].

Natural health specialists have used this ancient knowledge for years to treat their arthritis patients. More recently, researchers are confirming (and rheumatologists grudgingly accepting) that fish oils are a superb anti-inflammatory food.

A 1995 report from the research team of rheumatologist Dr. Joel Kremer found patients with rheumatoid arthritis who took fish oil capsules for at least eight weeks had less pain, fatigue, morning stiffness, swelling and far fewer tender joints than before. Some of his patients felt so comfortable with this natural treatment they threw away their pain pills[71]. Dr. Kremer's previous work revealed similar results with fish oil supplementation equal to one salmon dinner[72].

The omega-3 type oil in fatty fish, like sardines, herring, and trout, blocks prostaglandins that create inflammation. Instead, along with the help of vitamins E and C, and other nutrients, omega-3 fats push your body's biochemical pathways toward anti-inflammatory prostaglandins. Be patient with this approach as noticeable benefits take six weeks to three months[73].

Fish oil helps other inflammatory conditions like psoriasis[74], ulcerative colitis[75], a form of inflammatory bowel disease, and osteoarthritis where swelling is present[76]. The blood thinning property of fatty fish benefits those with atherosclerosis[70]. Even autoimmune diseases like multiple sclerosis and lupus respond to this simple, food-medicine[77].

Pick the Fattiest Fish for Your Arthritis

Unlike many foods you eat, the fattier your fish dinner, the better. To help you choose the juiciest, most inflammation-lowering fish for your meal, select dark, cold water types. They include:

Albacore tuna

American eel

*Anchovies

Bluefish

*Herring

*Mackerel

Pilchard

Rainbow trout

Russian sturgeon

Salmon

*Sardines

Sprat

Omega-3 oils are found in plants too such as soybeans, walnuts, and flax seeds[78].

*These fish should be avoided if you have gout as they are also high in purines. Other fish on the list can be served occasionally.

Recovery Food #2: Boosting Intake of Certain Vitamins and Minerals Benefits Most Cases of Arthritis or Gout

Mollie R. first had rheumatoid arthritis at age 45. Treatment began with aspirin, but the pain in Mollie's hands and wrists became so intolerable that a few months later her doctor began using steroids. After three years on corticosteroids, Mollie's face acquired a rounded, moon-like appearance, she felt constantly depressed and her condition had steadily deteriorated. Gradually, her knees and ankles also succumbed to arthritic pain. By age 49, Mollie could walk only with the aid of a cane. She consulted a second rheumatologist who urged surgery as the only alternative for her deteriorating left knee.

Finally, out of sheer frustration, Mollie went to a chiropractor who specialized in nutritional therapy. Instead of further drugs and surgery, the chiropractor ordered Mollie to eliminate all high-risk foods (our stressor foods) from her diet and to replace them with fresh fruits, vegetables, nuts, and seeds (our restorative foods). He especially recommended a liberal serving of what he called the "Seeds and Citrus Mix."

To make it, mix a large handful of hulled sunflower seeds with two tablespoonfuls of unhulled sesame seeds. Sprinkle with sliced kelp or dulse (seaweed available in health food stores) and add two tablespoons of brewer's yeast. Then eat the whole thing together with a large grapefruit or with two oranges. On alternate days, you can eat it with a large tomato or with two or three smaller ones.

Mollie alternated a spoonful of the seeds with a mouthful of citrus or tomatoes. From the day she first began to eat the mix, Mollie never looked back. Along with her dietary changes, she ceased taking all medication. The chiropractor also made her a heel lift that had her walking normally again with six weeks.

Rich in B-complex vitamins and vitamins A, C, D, and E, the seed-citrus combination is also packed with calcium, magnesium, manganese, zinc, and other anti-arthritic nutrients and enzymes. By her fiftieth birthday, Mollie was entirely free of all arthritic pain and stiffness.

In the five years since, she has had no serious arthritic flare-up, and each attack has been less severe and brief than the previous one. She stays regularly with the "Seeds and Citrus Mix" which she thoroughly enjoys. She finds that giving up the rich gremlin foods that she formerly ate is a small price to pay for her newfound freedom from pain and disablement.

Recovery Food #3: Old-time Remedy Becomes Hot New Drug

While browsing through a recent issue of Arthritis Today, a magazine put out by the Arthritis Foundation, we stumbled upon an advertisement for a pain-relieving cream containing a cayenne pepper extract. This is a perfect example of modern medicine rediscovering what herbalists have always known—food can be medicinal.

Ancient healers have rubbed hot peppers on painful body parts for hundreds of years. The active ingredient in hot peppers is capsaicin, which means "to bite" in Latin. It reduces achiness by lowering substance P, a neurotransmitter that activates inflammation in joints and relays painful sensations to your brain.

Various studies reveal that up to 80 percent of subjects with osteo or rheumatoid arthritis benefit from rubbing cayenne cream on their sore joints after only two weeks. Optimally, these creams are applied four times a day.

Eating these spicy peppers, including paprika also has its advantages. Like many brightly colored vegetables, hot peppers are loaded with antioxidant active carotenes, as well as vitamins C and A. Cayenne diminishes your chance of heart disease by reducing blood triglyceride and cholesterol levels. And contrary to popular belief hot peppers assist, not destroy, digestive function in people without ulcers[79].

Recovery Food #4: *Living on the Wild Side is Remarkably Therapeutic*

"Wild plants were our original vegetables," says Dr. Silena Heron, an expert herbalist and naturopathic doctor from Sedona, Arizona, "and several are still used both as herbal medicines and foods, especially in Europe."

Dr. Heron cultivates herbs for her patients and colleagues and acts as a professional botanical consultant. In her opinion, the most helpful arthritis herbs are dandelion (root and leaf), nettles, celery seeds, and alfalfa. Dandelion's reputation as an anti-gout medicine makes sense since it increases uric acid excretion. Toxins are flushed away when this weed exerts its diuretic action and stimulates the filtering liver.

Infamous stinging nettles are actually a pleasant tasting and nutritious addition to soups or other foods. (Cooking takes away nettle's sting.) They also act as a diuretic and increase joint circulation.

Celery seeds have diuretic and relaxing effects, both important components of arthritis treatment. Alfalfa, like nettles, is rich in vitamins, minerals, enzymes, and chlorophyll. While not well documented scientifically, alfalfa has a long tradition as a useful arthritis medicine.

All of these vegetable-herbs should be used consistently for several consecutive months for pain to significantly decrease.

Hunting in the Backyard

If you don't spray pesticides on your lawn, pick those pesky dandelions from your backyard and add the greens to a salad for both their bitter, digestive ability and pain relieving actions.

Dandelion roots and leaves can be dried for later use in a tea. Fresh dandelions can also be used.

For a superior spring tonic that will wake up your liver and spring-clean your body, take one teaspoon of dried dandelion leaf and add to one cup of hot water. Let steep for 15 minutes and drink. Three cups a day are fine for a month. If you want more dramatic effects for acute inflammation, up the herbal dose to one tablespoon per cup of water until symptoms fade.

To use the root, pulverize it in a coffee grinder or blender. Add boiling water to a thermos and scoop in an appropriate amount of powdered herb. Let sit for 40 minutes, filter, and serve. You can also boil the intact root in water for 30 minutes in order to loosen its medicinal ingredients.

Recovery Food #5: Five Years of Arthritic Pain Ends Abruptly When Herbert L. Switches to a Certain Breakfast Cereal

Soon after his fortieth birthday, Herbert L. was diagnosed as having rheumatoid arthritis of the right arm with degeneration of the spine. To kill the pain and reduce inflammation, his doctor prescribed 12 aspirins daily plus a periodic dosage of steroids. Herbert, who ran a plumbing business, often found the pain so intense that he took as many as 15 or even 20 aspirins daily. The aspirin caused severe stomach irritation. Yet nothing else helped.

That was until a knowledgeable aunt came to spend a vacation with Herbert and his wife. Although a self-taught amateur, the aunt was wise in the ways of nutrition. She was appalled by Herbert's diet, a seemingly endless round of rich meats, sausage, and cheeses with generous amounts of potato chips, white bread, cakes, pastries, and sugary desserts, all washed down with gallons of coffee and soda drinks.

By her second day, the aunt had persuaded Herbert to make a radical change in the way he ate. So great was his discomfort that Herbert reluctantly agreed to try it. Because his aunt correctly diagnosed a severe deficiency in B-complex vitamins, Herbert was to begin each day with a cereal rich in vitamins B_1, B_2, B_3, B_5, and B_6.

A Nutrient-Packed Arthritis Tonic That May Help End Pain for Good

For breakfast each morning, Herbert was to eat a bowl of cooked brown rice into which was mixed a large handful of wheat germ, two tablespoons of wheat bran, and two tablespoons of brewer's yeast. Blackstrap molasses was added for sweetening. Atop the cereal and eaten along with it were numerous chunks of fresh pineapple and honeydew or cantaloupe. There was also a small side dish of pecans and sunflower seeds. Herbert nibbled at the nuts and seeds between spoonfuls of the cereal and fruit.

What Herbert was getting turned out to be two bowls of nutritional dynamite fairly bursting with thiamine (B_1), riboflavin (B_2), niacin (B_3), pantothenic acid (B_5), and pyridoxine (B_6) along with a generous supply of natural vitamin C and enough fiber to thoroughly cleanse out his intestines and restore normal elimination.

Amazingly, Herbert began to feel better soon after his second breakfast with the new cereal. His aunt replaced the strong coffee with unlimited amounts of freshly-squeezed orange juice. She also urged Herbert to cease taking aspirin and any other drugs.

The pain Herbert dreaded never materialized. As the B-complex and C vitamins went to work to rebuild his collagen, to generate synovial fluid, and to stimulate his adrenal glands to produce more cortisone, Herbert felt increasingly cheerful and optimistic.

Although Herbert's pain and stiffness ended quite abruptly, complete recovery took considerably longer. But gradually, the symptoms tapered off and Herbert recovered full use and flexibility of his arm and back.

Herbert's speedy recovery should not surprise us. Tests have repeatedly shown that blood levels of B-complex and C vitamins in people with arthritis are often 75 percent lower than in healthy men and women. When rheumatologist Dr. William Kaufman treated 663 arthritis patients with niacinamide (B_3), almost all reported gains in overcoming joint stiffness, muscle weakness, and fatigue. Vitamin B_6 has also been found beneficial in relieving joint pain, especially in the hands.

A combination of vitamins C and B_6 (plus other B-complex vitamins) has been found to raise the threshold of immune response.

What this means is that an abundant supply of B-complex and C vitamins can reduce the pain and inflammation of rheumatoid and similar forms of arthritis.

Recovery Food #6: Everyday Spice Endowed with Endless Healing Potential

When you drink ginger ale or nibble on gingerbread cookies, did you know you're ingesting a medicinal spice? That's right! Ginger, embraced by traditional Ayurvedic doctors from India and Chinese medical healers, attacks arthritis pain from every angle.

It kills pain much the same way as cayenne does, by slashing substance P levels. Known throughout the ages as an anti-inflammatory medicine, modern experiments explain that this property is due to inhibition of pain producing prostaglandins. Too, ginger is a strong antioxidant ready to sweep away detrimental oxidants.

When poor digestion contributes to arthritis misery, ginger tea is the perfect intestinal tonic. It stimulates appetite, prevents gas and bloating, fights diarrhea and nausea, heals gastric ulcers, and even has antibiotic abilities. To top it off, ginger is rich in joint mending nutrients niacin and vitamin A[79].

K. C. Srivastava and T. Mustafa from Odense University in Denmark put ginger powder to the test. Of the 46 osteo and rheumatoid arthritic patients who used this food-medicine, three-quarters noticed an improvement in swelling and pain. Amounts taken and duration of treatment (three months to two and a half years) varied[80], but regular daily use is a place to start.

Many studies have used and found healing properties in ginger powder. However, like any plant product, fresh, whole ginger root is almost certainly more potent than the dried, ground-up variety.

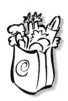

Raw Fresh Ginger Works Quickly to Relieve Arthritis Pain

The Danish researchers tell a story of a male patient from Asia who immigrated to Canada. When this gentlemen turned 50 years old, he was diagnosed with rheumatoid arthritis. He knew this disease would greatly restrict him from doing his job as an automechanic.

Drawing from his knowledge of Asian healing traditions, the patient began adding fresh, raw ginger root to his meals of lightly steamed vegetables and meat dishes. After one month, his painful and swollen joints got better. Two months later all pain and inflammation was gone.

More than a dozen years have passed since his diagnosis, and this Asian gentleman continues to enjoy ginger everyday in his meals. The Danish scientists report nodules have popped up on some of the patient's joints, but there is no pain or deformity, and the patient retains full use of his hands[80].

Recovery Food #7: Amazing Benefits from a Plant Extract Available at Any Health Food Store

Saponin, the naturally-occurring steroid-like compound found in a desert plant called yucca, is readily available in tablet form at almost any health food store. When yucca extract tablets were given to 212 arthritis patients in a study by Drs. Laga, Harris, and Bingham in California, approximately 66 percent reported at least some benefit and relief from pain and swelling.

The tablets contained dry yucca juice, a natural medicine used by Indian tribes for hundreds of years to relieve arthritis pain. By taking from 2–8 tablets per day, the yucca extract produces an effect similar to cortisone on arthritis-caused inflammation. Yet yucca is entirely safe, natural, and free of side effects.

For best results, you should take one tablet every four hours during the day (an average of four tablets daily). Larger, heavier people may take six or even eight tablets a day. Along with the yucca extract, you are advised to eat a liberal slice of avocado and a whole banana.

Alfalfa is another plant that contains saponin. In tests, alfalfa has also lowered cholesterol and reduced headaches and arthritis pain. Alfalfa is best taken as sprouts or as an herbal tea.

You can boost intake of saponin by using a fairly strong brew of alfalfa tea as a beverage. To prepare it, stew one ounce of untreated alfalfa seeds (identical to those used for sprouting) in 2 1/2 pints of water. Stir occasionally as it simmers for 30 minutes. Then strain out the seeds and drink up to 7 cups daily. Prepare a fresh brew every 24 hours.

Lorrie T. Uses Nature's Own Steroid to Reduce Her Swollen Joints

At 57, Lorrie T. had crippling rheumatoid arthritis pains in her hands and knees. She also suffered from diverticulosis and constipation so badly she could barely function. Her doctor had tried every type of medication but all Lorrie got was side effects.

On her 58th birthday, a friend advised Lorrie to change to a diet of natural foods and also to try taking yucca tablets. Exactly four days after starting, Lorrie began to go to the bathroom with unfailing regularity. A week later, her diverticulosis symptoms quietly faded away. Four weeks after that, her arthritis pains disappeared.

It took only another two months before Lorrie was up and about and moving as freely as she'd done 50 years before. At age 61, Lorrie now enjoys vigorous health and has had no hint of arthritis in the intervening three years.

Recovery Food #8: Nature's Analgesic Ends Pain from Rheumatoid Arthritis and Low Back Pain

Garlic, a common garden vegetable available in almost all supermarkets and in extract form at health food stores, contains selenium, a trace element which helps normalize the immune response.

When Japanese researchers tested garlic extract on patients with arthritis and low pack pain, 86 percent of the patients reported a noticeable improvement. None complained of side effects.

Dr. Satosi Kitahara, a Japanese professor of toxicology at Kumamoto University, has reportedly found that garlic extract aids in arthritis treatment by beefing up the immune system, soothing indigestion, acting as a diuretic, exerting its antioxidant abilities, and calming inflammation. If an intestinal infection is creating digestive grief or pathogenic germs are overcrowding your gut, garlic, with its natural antibiotic properties, is one solution.

Garlic's other natural therapeutic qualities include warding off cancer, protecting against strokes and heart disease, soothing feverish brows, easing nausea and vomiting, lowering blood cholesterol, diminishing high blood pressure, shedding surplus fat by hiking metabolic rate, and rejuvenating the entire body.

Although you can and should add garlic to any stew or similar dish when cooking, garlic capsules—some odorless—obtainable at most health food stores offer a more convenient way to take garlic twice daily.

For best results, take one garlic capsule twice each day. Supplements are best taken with a generous-sized helping of leafy green lettuce and a fresh, ripe tomato.

Onion, a cousin of garlic, is endowed with similar though milder powers.

Although garlic has been found most helpful for rheumatoid arthritis, it has also proved beneficial for both osteoarthritis and gout. When eating the clove, raw is more medicinal than cooked.

Recovery Food #9: Wonder Fruits That May Phase Out the Pain of Gouty Arthritis

A well-known Nature Cure clinic in the Southwest makes a point of serving half a pound of cherries twice daily to gout patients whenever the fruit is freshly available.

Their reasoning is based on the work of Dr. Ludwig N. Blair who, back in the 1940s, accidentally discovered that he could trigger a dramatic drop in his own blood uric acid level by eating half a pound or more of cherries each day. Although cherries are still the preferred fruit, subsequent experiments have shown that cherry juice is almost as effective.

Flavonoids such as procyanthocyandin provide cherries with their deep red hue, put the black and blues in blue and blackberries, and color other fruits like strawberries and cranberries. Like so many other phyto (plant) chemicals, procyanthocyandins are a Pandora's box of healing. Gout, osteo, and rheumatoid arthritis are helped by these flavonoids's anti-inflammatory actions, free radical scavenging, and ability to strengthen cartilage, tendons, and joints[81].

Here's another fascinating insight into cherries, the wonder fruit. Because the stalks of cherry plants (not the fruit) have been used as a diuretic in folk medicine, Hungarian researchers decided to test the anti-inflammatory capability of cherry stalk extract. What they found was the branches, as well as the fruit, of a cherry plant reduce swelling[82].

Unless organically grown, all berries should be thoroughly rinsed and washed to help remove any traces of pesticide before eating.

Whenever cherries are available, you may eat from 1/2–1 pound daily. Other fruits can be eaten alone or mixed together in a tasty fruit salad.

Recovery Food #10: A Natural Health Booster That Renews and Recharges the Whole Body

Eight years ago, her doctor told Sue M. that she had a severe case of osteoarthritis and that it would become increasingly worse with the passing of years. He told her to rest and relax, to avoid all vigorous activity and to take aspirin to relieve the pain and inflammation.

Sue did none of these things. Instead, she phoned the director of a well-known arthritis clinic in the Southwest and asked for his advice. Among the dietary changes suggested was a snack to be taken twice daily.

Each mid-morning and mid-afternoon, in place of her usual coffee break, Sue was to eat a large, fresh apple with an equal amount of fresh, raw carrot. The two were to be sliced up in a bowl and sprinkled with chopped kelp or dulse (seaweeds obtainable in health food stores).

Although her other dietary changes seemed beneficial, Sue felt most enthusiastic about the carrot-apple-seaweed snack. Each time she ate the snack, an hour or so later the stiffness and ache in her spine and knees became slightly less intense. Gradually, day by day, the arthritis symptoms subsided. Three months after she first began the twice-daily snack, Sue realized she was completely free of arthritis pain.

Although Sue has experienced an occasional return of pain since, each time it was briefer and less severe than before. Throughout the intervening eight years, Sue has not once missed her carrot-apple-seaweed snack. She plays tennis every day and is able to run, walk, swim, or ride a bicycle with ease.

To prepare the snack, rinse and scrub the apple well before serving if it is not organic. But under no circumstances peel the apple. Apple skins are rich in the fiber pectin, one of nature's most effective dietary cleansing agents. Tests have shown that pectin "scrubs" cholesterol out of the arteries and keeps blood vessels youthful and flexible. Pectin also moistens and helps eliminate any hard, dry feces in the colon.

Raw carrots are rich in calcium, magnesium, manganese, and vitamin A and help normalize the actions of the liver and pancreas. Carrots also exert a profound and lasting improvement in elimination and colon action. In a study reported in the *American Journal of Clinical Nutrition* (September 1979) when researchers at the Western General Hospital in Edinburgh, Scotland fed seven ounces of raw carrot to five healthy people each day for three weeks, their blood cholesterol levels dropped by 11 percent. Their stool weights also increased by 25 percent while bile acid excretion in the stools rose by 50 percent.

Recovery Food #11: How the Coloring in Curry Cuts-down on Pain

If you like curry, then you're already eating a terrific anti-arthritis food. Turmeric, the spice that gives curry and prepared mustard their bright orange-yellow color, quells swollen joints, protects the liver, acts as an antioxidant, increases digestive enzyme secretion, and prevents stomach upset.

Curcumin, turmeric's medicinally strong pigment, is often used in place of the milder pure turmeric spice. Dr. John O'Hearne, associate clinical professor of family practice at the University of Colorado in Boulder, uses curcumin mixed with another natural substance called bromelain to treat patients with lupus. This natural therapy is such an effective anti-inflammatory agent that one of his patients was able to kick his daily 1000 mg steroid habit for curcumin instead[83]. Not only is curcumin (or turmeric) without serious side effects, but unlike drugs it contains vitamins and minerals for your joints.

Turmeric can be sprinkled liberally on food to curtail swelling and pain, or you can partake of your favorite curried dishes. A traditional treatment from India calls for turmeric powder mixed with lime juice and applied as a poultice to aching, inflamed joints. You can also purchase curcumin supplements from the health food store.

Recovery Food #12: A Mineral-Rich Natural Oil Helps Carole R. Phase Out Years of Arthritis Pain

The story of Carole R.'s rheumatoid arthritis reads like a textbook case history. It began with a small swelling in the middle joint of her right index finger. Soon, the entire finger became swollen. Carole could not bend it. Three months later, all the fingers of her right hand were painful and swollen. Pain appeared next in her ankles, neck, shoulders, wrists, and elbows. As she got out of bed each morning, the aching and stiffness in these joints was almost unbearable.

Carole's doctor gave her the usual X-rays and tests for rheumatoid factor, uric acid level, sedimentation rate, blood count, and urinalysis. When the results came in, Carole was given the standard textbook verdict: "You have a severe case of rheumatoid arthritis. There is no known cure. Take plenty of rest and relaxation. Avoid strenuous activity. Eat plenty of protein. And take aspirin to relieve the tenderness and inflammation."

Just as medical textbooks predict, Carole began a life of crippling pain, disablement, and deformity that was to last for three further agony-filled years.

That it did not last longer was entirely due to the arrival in Carole's town of a doctor of naturopathy who had been trained at a Nature Cure clinic specializing in arthritis. Completely disenchanted by now with medicine's failure to relieve her suffering, Carole made an appointment with the naturopathic doctor on the first day he opened his office.

The naturopathic doctor diagnosed Carole as suffering from faulty calcium metabolism. Her vitamin D intake was so low that her body was unable to absorb the calcium in her food. As a result, calcium was being leached out of her bones and teeth and forming into deposits that restricted movement in her afflicted joints.

Among the naturopathic doctor's advice was a recommendation to take a tablespoon of cod liver oil twice each day; a 200 year old English tradition for rheumatism and gout[71]. The naturopathic doctor explained that this natural fish oil supplies biologically active vitamin D that is needed before the body can utilize calcium in food.

Cod liver oil is also rich in vitamin A which is believed to help normalize immune system function and to stimulate regeneration of damaged tissue. Like other fish oils, it's also full of eicosapentaenoic acid, the stuff of omega-3 fats that calms inflammation.

For several weeks, Carole noticed no difference. Then one morning, she detected a new flexibility in her normally stiff right elbow.

The following morning, the fingers of her right hand seemed more mobile than usual. Day by day, the stiffness slowly faded from her joints. Once she could move her joints without pain, Carole could feel the calcium deposits cracking and creaking. To limber up her joints, the naturopathic doctor advised Carole to do lots of easy stretching and bending movements.

This therapy was so effective that three months after first taking cod liver oil, Carole was able to walk normally and to swing her arms freely over her head.

In the intervening years, during which Carole has never once missed her ration of cod liver oil, her condition has constantly improved. Today, her bone density is completely normal and she has no trace of either arthritis or osteoporosis.

Recovery Food #13: Bitter Medicinal-Food Helps Digestion and Arthritis

What do mustard greens, escarole, watercress, and chamomile all have in common? They're what we call "bitters" because of their bitter, astringent taste. It's this biting flavor that gets your saliva and gastric juices flowing for better digestion.

Natural health practitioners recommend these bitter foods especially for people with low stomach acid. Results from a 1993 Swedish study indicated that 32 percent of the patients they tested with rheumatoid arthritis had low or no stomach acid. Half of these individuals were also plagued by intestinal bacterial overgrowth[84].

A marvelous way to get the living enzymes you need and stimulate digestion at the same time is to feast on a raw vegetable salad that includes endive or other bitter lettuce.

Recovery Food #14: Dramatic Results from a Gentle Curative Agent

During the late 1970s, the U.S. Department of Agriculture conducted a study in which several different types of animals were raised on a diet rich in yogurt. Results revealed that all the animals fed yogurt grew larger, stronger, and healthier than comparable control animals fed a normal diet. Similar studies since on both animals and humans have convinced many biologists of yogurt's wide reaching health benefits.

Despite containing cholesterol, yogurt actually lowers serum cholesterol levels when eaten regularly. Its calcium and acid content have also proved extremely beneficial in numerous cases of gouty arthritis.

To be of therapeutic value, yogurt must contain *Lactobacillus acidophilus* or other healthful micro-organisms that crowd out unfriendly bacteria that afflict the intestinal tract. As a result, yogurt has special properties for restoring intestinal health, a vital step in recovering from arthritic disease.

If you prefer, try one of the many acidophilus or other beneficial micro-organisms available in pill form. Some of these supplements need refrigeration.

Not all commercial yogurts contain acidophilus but most health food stores carry brands that do. Or you can easily make your own yogurt with acidophilus starter and a yogurt maker.

A Substitute If You Cannot Tolerate Milk

Researchers believe that fermented foods like yogurt can be tolerated by many people with a food sensitivity to milk. Yogurt bacteria apparently digest some of the lactose (milk sugar) in milk, thus transforming it into a tolerated food for those with lactose sensitivity.

During the same USDA studies, when control rats were fed equal amounts of milk fortified with massive doses of vitamins, the yogurt-fed rats still outperformed them.

One arthritis clinic has experimented with yogurt as a restorative food and found encouraging results. The recommended amount is 16 ounces of plain, non-fat acidophilus yogurt divided into three portions and served as a snack three times daily. (That is, a full pound is eaten each day.) The yogurt must be free of any additional sugar, gelatin, flavoring, or additives. If preferred, a small amount of honey or fresh fruit or nuts may be used for flavor. Or, as in the Balkans, yogurt can be eaten with whole grain bread.

Observations have shown that this restorative food is even more effective when combined with 15 minutes of daily sunbathing. Sunbathing is nature's way of providing vitamin D. If this is not possible, consider taking two tablespoons of cod liver oil daily or the same amount in capsule form, or a vitamin D pill (200 I.V. daily).

Walter W., a patient at the arthritis clinic, had suffered with severe gout symptoms in his hands, feet, and knees during each of the previous five winters. During January and February each year, his uric acid level was as high as 13 mg/dl.

After spending the month of September at the clinic and becoming accustomed to eating the yogurt snack three times each day on a permanent basis, Walter was completely free of gout throughout the following winter. He has since continued to take the yogurt snacks regularly every day and has had no recurrence of gout at any time since.

Recovery Food #15: The Tropical Fruit Treatment

Nothing tastes more delicious than an exquisitely ripe pineapple on a hot summer's day. This flavorful South American fruit is also the source of bromelain, a protein-digesting enzyme with anti-inflammatory and digestive talents.

Back in 1956, a Philadelphia dentist reported that bromelain diminished pain and swelling in his patients suffering from multiple dental impactions[85]. One year later bromelain's arthritis helping abilities were first reported. Since then researchers have kept busy investigating this natural inflammation fighter, documented in more than 200 scientific papers[86]. Natural health care providers utilize bromelain as a digestive enzyme replacement, to ease pain, and increase absorption of both natural and synthetic medicines[87].

Papaya, with its protein-digesting enzyme papain, along with pineapple, can be added to a pre-meal fruit salad. Or mix a tropical fruit cocktail as a during-meal digestive aid. Papaya must be on the green side of ripe to garner the most papain. Bromelain and papain tablets are also available from your local health food store.

Recovery Food #16: How a Common Weed Brings Arthritic Relief

For thousands of years Greeks, Romans, and Egyptians used mint to pacify indigestion, treat colds, and erase headaches.

Centuries later, we rely on menthol lozenges, derived form mint, for sore throats and colds, and eat peppermint candy after dinner so our stomachs settle easier. Peppermint herbal tea is a fine conclusion to meals for those with arthritis.

Aching joints and muscles quieten down when peppermint oil is gently rubbed on them. Menthol, peppermint's main volatile oil, relieves pain by first cooling the skin then warming it up. By all means use the oil of this common weed for temporary comfort from pain. But beware: too much oil may cause a skin rash.

Recovery Food #17: *The Traditional Chinese Medicine View of Food and Arthritis*

Dr. Ilene Dahl, a licensed acupuncturist from Concord, California, says traditional Chinese medical doctors use arthritis symptoms to decide what foods their patients should eat. This is what she has to say.

"For cold type arthritis, which is worse in cold weather and better with heat or hot applications, eat the following foods:

Black beans	Grapes	Parsnips
Chicken	Green onions	Pepper
Garlic	Lamb	Sesame seeds
Ginger	Mustard greens	Spicy foods

Avoid cold, raw foods.

For damp type arthritis, which is worse with damp, rainy weather and sometimes better with heat and primarily better with dryness, eat these foods:

Barley	Millet	Sweet rice wine
Beans (especially red)	Mustard greens (with meals)	
Cornsilk tea		

Avoid cold, raw foods including dairy products and tofu.

For heat-type arthritis which usually has more inflammation and a sensation of heat, and is better with cool applications, use these foods:

Cabbage	Fresh vegetables	Soybean sprouts
Dandelion	Mung beans	Winter melon
Fresh fruits	Soybeans	

Avoid spicy foods, alcohol, green onions, and cinnamon[88].

Recovery Food #18: Why the Seaweed-Eating Japanese Seldom Got Gout

Until the mid-1960s gout was almost unknown among working class Japanese. For decades preceding the early 1960s, the average Japanese lived largely on tofu, fish, seaweed, and brown rice.

Then came a new affluence that changed the diet of even the poorest classes. Nowadays, brown rice is considered "peasant food." This nutrient-rich whole grain has been replaced by denatured polished rice which contains little else but empty calories. Along with the new affluence has come white flour (called "American flour"), deep fried foods, rich meats, and a variety of pickled junk foods, sugar drinks, and candy.

Not surprisingly, by the early 1970s, Japan experienced a skyrocketing surge in almost every degenerative disease including not only gout and arthritis but heart disease, cancer, diabetes, and hypertension. Previously, when most Japanese had lived on a low-fat diet of natural, largely high-fiber foods, these diseases were approximately one tenth as common as in the U.S.

Recovery Food #19: One More Plus for the Traditional Japanese Diet

The shiitake, or Japanese forest mushroom, is a cherished and high-priced delicacy. Its mild smoky flavor makes soups more tempting; its lentinan and vitamins make it a worthy addition to your arthritis program.

For years Japanese researchers have probed this mealtime mushroom to see what makes it so healing. Lentinan is the polysaccharide found in shiitakes that bolster body defenses against cancer, infections, and possibly autoimmune conditions like rheumatoid arthritis[72].

If you're lucky and find fresh shiitake mushrooms in your local market, pick ones with firm flesh and caps that are still slightly closed, for it is under the cap where healing spores lie. Fragrant shiitake mushrooms mean more flavor, too, for your soups and casseroles. For those who must settle for dried shiitakes, sold in health food and grocery stores, and specialty Asian shops, soak the caps three to four hours before using. Discard the stems, then add both caps and soaking water to whatever dish you're preparing.

Recovery Food #20: The Japanese Beverage That Curtails Swelling

What's a Japanese meal without green tea, the beverage with a medicinal punch? Both black and green teas originate from the plant *Camellia sinensis*. Yet because green tea is only lightly steamed before it's sold, it retains most of its oxidant-opposing polyphenols. Arthritic joints are riddled with these harmful oxidants.

Other arthritis advantages to green tea include its purported anti-inflammatory effects and digestive promoting properties.

The downside to green tea is, like its black tea cousin, it contains caffeine. If this bothers you, drink decaffeinated green tea before a meal, available at both grocery and health food stores.

A Medicinal Diet for Arthritic Disease

Many nutritionists believe that it was their diet of brown rice, tofu, and seaweed that kept the Japanese almost entirely free of gout in earlier times. This belief has spread to several arthritis clinics and health resorts in Europe where brown rice is used as part of the medicinal diet to treat heart disease, hypertension, and arthritis.

But you don't need to visit a European spa to include brown rice, seaweed, and tofu in your diet. Brown rice, preferably organically grown, is widely available in almost every food store along with seaweeds from Japan. Alternatively, you may use less expensive American seaweeds like kelp or dulse.

Tofu, a cheese-like curd made from soybeans, is also now available in most larger supermarkets and health food stores. Tempeh, the same as tofu but with the soybeans added back in, is a meatier alternative. These and other soy foods are the largest dietary supply of saponins, steroid-like substances that help arthritic joints recuperate.

To enjoy the same beneficial diet that the Japanese once had, build two or three meals weekly around a liberal helping of brown rice. Add nothing to the rice but water. Atop the rice serve an assortment of lightly steamed vegetables including vitamin C rich Brussels sprouts, broccoli, turnips, cabbage, pineapple, and seaweed, all flavored with garlic. If you prefer, you may prepare the vegetables in a wok.

Some people prefer to cook tofu together with the vegetables because this bland tasting food tends to soak up other flavors. Some add tofu after cooking. You may also sprinkle chopped seaweed or zesty spices on the vegetables after cooking.

For anyone who tests allergic to corn, oats, potatoes, or other staples, brown rice is a wonderful anti-arthritic alternative.

Recovery Food #21: Mother (Nature) Has the Last Word

"Eat your fruits and vegetables!" This is the mothers of the world (and Mother Nature) speaking—and we agree!

Americans are terribly lax when it comes to eating their daily recommended allotment of five to seven servings of produce a day. Only 20 percent are capable of doing so; less than 10 percent even know this is important[89]. But if you have arthritis, it's even more vital that you load up on those antioxidant powerhouses.

Individuals with low serum antioxidant levels, say Finnish scientists, are at higher risk of developing rheumatoid arthritis[90]. Antioxidants protect both arthritic and gouty joints from tissue destroying free radical molecules.

Of course, fresh fruits and vegetables also carry with them vitamins, minerals, enzymes, fiber, and who knows what else, absolutely vital for good health.

Chapter 15

Beating Arthritis with Weight-Reducing Foods

Statistics show that most people with gout or osteoarthritis are overweight. Surplus poundage is a major reason why osteoarthritis develops. Excessive body weight simply overburdens the weight-bearing joints in the spine, hips, and knees. Under the stress of this continual weight, the protective cartilage in the joint loses its elasticity and wears away, exposing the bones in the joint to grate painfully against each other.

Cartilage breaks down under excessive weight more easily when it is deficient in essential nutrients. Nutritional deficiency is almost standard in anyone who lives on a diet of stressor foods. stressor foods are frequently responsible for excessive weight. So stressor foods are a basic contributor to osteoarthritis.

Gout is a disease made worse by frequent indulgence in foods rich in purines (the basic component of uric acid). High-fat foods also disrupt purine metabolism and promote gout. Hence people who eat these foods often become overweight.

Once pain and inability to move appear, victims of both diseases are less likely to keep their weight down by activity and movement.

Both diseases can be greatly benefited by a change in eating habits and exercise that leads to weight loss. In fact, records show that for symptoms to completely disappear, a patient must restore his or her weight to normal.

257

In case you're thinking in terms of a fad diet, relax! Seldom do any of the crash diets you read about lead to permanent weight reduction. The safe, natural way to shed surplus pounds, and to keep them off for good, has already been described in this book.

It simply amounts to eating only restorative foods and eating them the 65-20-15 way.

Losing Weight While You Continue to Eat All You Want

How can eating lead to weight loss?

Because restorative foods are mostly low in fat and calories and high in enzymes and fiber. Living foods like fresh fruits and vegetables all contain enzymes which aid digestion.

Among the many doctors who have praised the benefits of low fat, high fiber natural foods is Dr. Neil Solomon. While on staff at Johns Hopkins Hospital, Baltimore, Dr. Solomon reportedly said that most metabolic disorders can be reversed with a low fat diet. Virtually all degenerative diseases are metabolic disorders and, as nutritionists have discovered, many can be permanently reversed by changing to a diet of Restorative Foods.

So powerful are the effects of a diet low in fat and high in fiber that many vegetarians are able to eat plentiful meals without ever adding weight. Several studies have shown that when at least 80 percent of the diet consists of fresh, uncooked fruits and vegetables, the fiber content is so high that the body doesn't absorb all the calories (remember fiber isn't absorbed). Fiber keeps you full longer, yet allows food to pass quickly through your GI tract and prevent constipation.

So while you're heaping your dinner plate with these high-fiber low-fat restorative foods go back for seconds. That deprived, hungry feeling you usually experience on a reducing diet will be gone. You're left instead with the full satisfaction and knowledge that you've fed your body the best quality nutrients.

Weight-Reducing Foods

This means that a diet of fresh fruits and vegetables with whole grains is the most effective way to restore normal weight. Provided you follow the 65-20-15 formula, you can eat all the restorative foods you wish without counting calories, though it's best to eat only when hungry.

If you are overweight, you will gradually lose weight. If underweight, you will gradually gain weight. Because genetic make-up also determines body type, "normal" weight varies between individuals with some slightly thinner or heavier than others.

To ensure a natural, healthful return to your optimum weight, 65 percent of your diet must consist of complex carbohydrates; 20 percent of calories can consist of fat; and 15 percent of complete protein. For more rapid weight loss, we suggest avoiding nuts, seeds, and avocados and replacing them with protein-rich soybeans and other beans, both sprouted and cooked. As soon as your weight normalizes, you can go back to nuts, seeds, and avocados—excellent sources of essential fatty acids.

Adding bran to conventional food does increase fiber and improve regularity. But it does not ensure weight loss and may even deter mineral absorption. By contrast, a diet that consists exclusively of high-fiber foods requires extensive chewing. You will feel full and satisfied long before you can overeat. By eating restorative foods the 65-20-15 way, your food is so bulky you seldom feel hungry.

To shed weight, all you need do is to follow the nutritional therapy described in this book for recovery from arthritis. By cutting out all stressor foods, you eliminate most foods high in fat. And by undertaking a two-week cleansing program, you can lose as much as five pounds right away.

Shed Fat While the Body Purifies Itself

Cleansing is one way to begin melting off pounds. While cleansing, excess feces are removed and the intestines cleaned out while the body feeds off its own fat cells.

Before cleansing, be sure to study Chapter 5 in detail, especially the section entitled, "Who should not undertake the purification technique."

If you are under medical treatment for any condition that might be affected by fasting or cleansing or a change in diet, you should consult your doctor first.

Cleansing is a wonderful kick-off to losing excess weight. Staying within proper guidelines, you can cleanse or fast periodically for example 1–2 days every month, staying with restorative foods in between. By following this eating program, most overweight people should be able to lose at least two pounds a week safely and naturally.

Through healthy eating and periodic cleansing, your taste buds wake up to the full flavor of restorative foods. After a few weeks of living foods, most people are turned off by sweet and fatty junk foods. As long as you continue to eat restorative foods the 65-20-15 way, the surplus weight should never return.

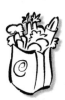 **Anna J. Shrinks Away Fat and Loses Her Arthritis**

According to standard height and weight tables, Anna J. should have weighed 130 pounds. But at age 55 she actually weighed 180. The burden of carrying around this surplus poundage caused such distress in her knees and hips that severe osteoarthritis set in. Gradually, the pain spread into her upper spine, and her shoulders became almost too stiff to move.

Anna knew that losing weight was her only hope, but she was simply unable to count calories or to diet.

One morning, she woke to find the pain in her hips had spread into her groin and down the insides of her thighs. She could barely shuffle around the house.

"It was just too much," Anna said. "That was my moment of truth. I decided then and there that I was going to take charge of my body and I was going to get well."

Anna enrolled at a natural hygiene health school in the next state. The doctor was aghast at her diet. Almost all of Anna's meals consisted of sugar and fat.

Anna was placed on a natural foods eating program. This meant cleansing two days a month followed by fresh foods like raw fruits and vegetables, beans, whole grains, and fish the rest of the time.

In a single month, Anna lost ten pounds and she felt sufficiently confident to continue the program at home. Another month of the program brought her weight down to 160.

As the pounds melted away, Anna felt better every day. The pain in her thighs and groin disappeared. She could move her spine and shoulders freely again. And discomfort was steadily diminishing in her knees and hips.

Anna lost her last 10 pounds on restorative foods alone. As the final pounds disappeared, she was able to do housework again and she began taking daily walks.

"I had to buy an entire new wardrobe," she said. "I went down from a size eighteen and a half to a size twelve."

That was many years ago. Anna still has the same trim figure and she is totally active and fit. How has she managed to stay on restorative foods?

"At the clinic I learned that natural foods like fruits, vegetables, nuts, and seeds are compatible with the human digestive system. But man cannot eat refined foods or foods high in fats without eventually becoming sick.

"Now that I'm well, I intend to stay that way. As far as I'm concerned, any kind of processed food is not fit for human consumption. I wouldn't eat any of those junkier foods for a million dollars."

An Eating Technique That Shrinks Your Waistline

If you're eating natural low-fat foods, your body will stop losing pounds once you reach your ideal weight. Exercise, even short walks, is vital to achieve this.

You can prevent much weight gain by eating earlier in the day. The U.S. Army Research and Development Command discovered that the earlier in the day you eat, the less fat you are likely to gain.

The explanation? Calories eaten before 11 a.m. are burned up during the day before they can turn into fat. But calories eaten later in the day, especially in the evening, turn into fat overnight.

To capitalize on this phenomenon, have your largest and heaviest meal for breakfast and schedule it early—as soon as you get up if possible. Make lunch your second heaviest meal and schedule it, too, as early as possible. Then eat lightly through the rest of the day.

Weight loss can be speeded up still more by using the mini-meal routine described in Chapter 16.

How to Stop Using Food for Solace

Are you one of those people who eat too much because of what is eating you? If so, whenever you head for the refrigerator, stop and ask yourself why you are about to eat. Are you using food to smoothe the stress of anxiety, boredom, loneliness, or feeling unhappy, unwanted, and unloved?

The solution here is to make a list of alternative pleasures, each of which is readily available and easy to do. For example, you might make love, listen to music, take a drive, go fishing, paint a picture, see a movie, read a novel, or do something physically active if you are able.

Whenever you feel the urge to eat, sample an alternative pleasure instead. Try to disassociate eating with pleasures like drinking, reading, or listening to music or watching TV or a movie. Never eat during these activities. Make eating an entirely separate activity.

For months following her divorce, Georgia R. would head for the refrigerator and load up on ice cream, pie, cookies, and sodas. Georgia's inevitable gain in weight finally brought on osteoarthritic-like pain in her knees. A psychologist friend suggested she find a substitute pleasure that brought more solace than compulsive eating.

Georgia had always wanted to paint. So she bought materials and took lessons in watercolor. Whenever she feels down, instead of heading for the refrigerator, she takes her easel and starts to paint. This motivational therapy worked so well for Georgia that over a 12-month period, her weight gradually dropped back to normal and her knees are pain-free once more.

Enjoy Life and Stay Thin

This might be a good place to mention the powerful benefits of movement and activity.

Once you have recovered sufficiently to move freely without pain, you should begin regular activity that involves gentle and easy yet progressive movements. The bending and stretching positions of yoga and the gentle, flowing movements of Tai Chi (a form of oriental martial arts) are perfect for restoring flexibility to once afflicted joints.

As recovery progresses, begin regular daily walks and such enjoyable activities as dancing, bicycling, or swimming. Many of the people in our case histories took immediate advantage of their ability to move again by becoming very active. Activity complements the health-restoring powers of nutrition and helps maintain the entire organism in optimum health. It enhances immunity, aids digestion, and prevents weight gain.

So use your body to enjoy life and to keep your weight down. Dance, play tennis or golf (without a cart), go canoeing or for bicycle rides, grow your own fruits and vegetables, or join an adult fitness club. Once you take up the active life, it's next to impossible to put on weight again or to get arthritis.

Chapter **16**

New Ways to Eat

Away Arthritis

So far in this book, we've been talking about WHAT we eat—food and nutrition. But HOW we eat—the very act of eating itself—also plays a major role in recovery from arthritis. Some cases of arthritic disease may actually be aggravated more by *how* we eat than by *what* we eat.

For example, you can greatly reduce exposure to allergy foods by rotating your diet and by eating mini-meals instead of the usual three "squares" a day. (Remember the 3-S rule: *several, small, simple meals.*) And you can often improve digestion (and reduce risk of arthritis) by using food to restore intestinal health.

By improving the way you eat, as well as what you eat, your arthritis therapy becomes more holistic.

 How to Eat Allergy Foods Safely Again

You may not have to stop eating all allergy foods permanently. The digestive diet plan helps as does adding more variety to your diet, so that servings of allergy foods are spaced farther apart. You can probably start to eat most of these foods again after a few weeks of abstinence.

The fact is that most of us simply don't eat the variety of foods that we should. Experiments have proved that when the body is in optimum health balance and free of all nutritional stress, we will naturally choose foods containing the nutrients we need.

But once the body's mechanisms are distorted by stressor foods or we're tired or tense, we choose comfort foods like sugar and fats that temporarily uplifts us and contribute to ill health.

Instead of eating a wide assortment of foods, we avoid diversification and keep on eating the same foods over and over. Most people eat only 12–16 different foods. As we continually eat large and frequent amounts of just a few foods, we may even crave them.

Ease of preparation also guides people to eat, say, a candy bar which is immediately available instead of waiting 30 minutes to bake some vegetables. If physical activity is restricted by arthritis, our choice of foods may be narrowed even more by inability to move around and shop.

Thus we continue to eat a relatively few foods, and often eat a single food several times a day. Our modern trucking industry allows us to keep these same foods on the table every day of the year.

But in nature, foods change with the season. Primitive peoples found a variety of alternative and different foods that provided a perfect nutritional balance.

By adding more variety to your diet and eating more kinds of different foods, you may very well be able to once again begin eating certain foods to which you have an allergy. This is possible because there are two types of food allergies.

- *Fixed Allergies* are innate and may be caused by a genetic intolerance. They will always be with you. No matter how long you abstain from a food or how little you may eat, an allergic reaction will always occur.

- *Cyclical Allergies* are an acquired rejection response that develops as the result of distorted digestion, and nutritional or other stress.

Fortunately, cyclical allergies are by far the more common. The only way to ascertain which type you have is to abstain from an allergenic food for several weeks, then to challenge it. If no reaction occurs, it may be a cyclical allergy or no allergy at all.

The Astounding Rotation System for Overcoming Allergies

After an abstinence of six weeks or more, cyclical allergy foods can be reintroduced into the diet provided that:

- You eat no allergy food more often than once very 5 days.
- You eat no allergy food from any one family more often than every other day.
- Not more than one allergy food should be eaten on any one day.

Let's say you have cyclical allergies to wheat, corn, veal, chicken, and peanuts. After abstaining from these foods for six weeks, you become temporarily desensitized to them.

Within the guidelines just described, you may then try reintroducing each of these foods back into your diet. For example, you could eat wheat on Monday, veal on Tuesday, corn on Wednesday, chicken on Thursday, and peanuts on Friday. In this way, the two grass family cereals (corn and wheat) are spaced two days apart. (Food families are listed in Chapter 8.)

The rest of your food doesn't have to be on a 5-day rotational basis. You can eat non-allergenic foods more often. But to discourage any possible tendency to future intolerances, it is wise to rotate your foods and to eat as many widely different foods as you can.

Some people may have multiple allergies to as many as ten or even 15 different foods. If you have this many cyclical allergies, you must still space them out so that only one allergy food is eaten each day. Should you try to eat normal-sized helpings of two or more allergenic foods in one day, the total allergenic exposure could well be sufficient to trigger an arthritis flare-up.

If you desire to eat two allergenic foods in one day, then eat only half a serving of each.

Some apparent food allergies aren't true immune reactions. They are actually intolerances or sensitivities due to other factors. That is why repairing your gastrointestinal tract, one reason for food intolerances, may allow you to consume a previously sensitive food.

A *Sample Five-Day Rotation Menu*

Here is a sample menu in which the five allergy foods (in capitals) are rotated on a 5-day basis. Treat between meal snacks the same way. All foods listed can be prepared or combined any way you wish for each meal.

Day	Breakfast	Lunch	Dinner

1	Cantaloupe
	Brown rice
	Soy milk, almonds,
	  raisins & honey
		Vegetable salad
		Yogurt
		WHOLE WHEAT
		  BREAD
			Vegetable salad
			Baked haddock
			Potatoes, peas,
			  parsnips & onions

2	Apple Pear Oatbran Yogurt	Vegetable salad VEAL Baked potatoes Green beans	Vegetable salad Baked cod Brown rice Steamed vegeta- bles Navy beans

3	Frantic Fruit
	  Smoothie (*See
	  recipe on page* 197)
		Vegetable salad
		Soybeans
		PEANUTS
		Sunflower and
		  sesame seeds
		Mixed nuts
			Vegetable salad
			Baked haddock
			Rutabagas
			Turnips
			Beans
			Peas
			Onions

4	Pineapple Oatmeal Cashews	Vegetable salad Baked haddock CORN Green beans	Salmon Vegetable salad Wok-prepared vegetables
5	Frantic Fruit Smoothie	Vegetable salad CHICKEN Baked potato Peas	Vegetable salad Vegetable soup Sweet potatoes White beans Onions

Although the menu contains more cooked vegetables than is perhaps ideal, it still meets the 65-20-15 guidelines because of the large vegetable salads that precede each lunch and dinner. Salad vegetables would be varied as much as possible to include sprouts, tomatoes, and other desired vegetables.

As restorative foods rebuild total health, including digestion, sensitivities to cyclical allergy foods may gradually disappear altogether. But this can take a year or more. Meanwhile, use a rotational menu to space out cyclical allergy foods so that you can continue to eat them without triggering a rejectivity response.

The Reverend C. Eats Allergy Foods Safely Once More

The Reverend C. had suffered from rheumatoid arthritis since his early fifties. When he retired at 65, he took time off to enroll at a naturally oriented arthritis clinic. There he fasted for five days and tested allergy-positive to sugar, corn, oats, beef, milk, and cheese.

Recovery was gradual but steady. Three months later, Reverend C. was able to walk for several miles and to swim and ride a bicycle.

After phoning the arthritis clinic, Reverend C. was advised to try reintroducing corn and oats back into his diet. Since both were grass family cereals, he was advised to eat each once every four days and to eat them only on alternate days. This meant that during a 4-day cycle, Reverend C. ate corn the first day and oats on the third day.

By carefully observing this rotational technique, Reverend C. found that he could eat two ears of corn on the first day and a large bowl of oatmeal on the third day without any hint of arthritis symptoms.

Poor Digestion May Be Causing Arthritis

Poor digestion is often at the bottom of delayed food allergies. Almost everyone with severe or multiple food allergies suffers from some degree of gastrointestinal trouble—especially apparent whenever they eat the allergenic food.

Strangely, however, instead of the allergy causing poor digestion, it is probably the other way around.

Faulty chewing and improper eating can lead to incomplete digestion. Add to this, poor food selections, emotional and mental stress, drugs, and other gut disruptions, and you have trouble. When food is not fully digested, the number of partly digested food particles increases. When this load of particles is absorbed into the bloodstream, they overwhelm the liver and may set off an immune response that triggers joint pain. Thus the poorer the digestion, the greater the risk of rheumatoid and similar forms of arthritis.

In any event, you can benefit both your arthritis and your digestion by learning the rules of successful eating.

Improper mastication and faulty digestion are the usual causes of bloating, excess gas, heartburn, indigestion, and many cases of constipation and diarrhea. When enzymes are low, as in cooked and refined foods, food may be poorly absorbed and nutrient value is lower.

By obeying the six rules of successful digestion below, you can speed your recovery from arthritis.

What we've been talking about so far in this book concerns food and nutrition. The rules below govern the act of eating.

Six Rules for Eating Away Gout and Arthritis

Rule #1: Never overeat or stuff yourself. Avoid large meals. Eat mini-meals instead.

The smaller your meals, the less your digestion is stressed and the more stable is your blood sugar. This reduces your risk of food allergies and arthritic disease. Five to six frequent meals are ideal provided they are small.

A two-year study of 4,057 people aged 20 and over conducted by Dr. Allen B. Nichols at the University of Michigan revealed that eating larger meals can be as dangerous to the heart and blood vessels as a high-fat diet. Whenever a large meal is eaten, the body is stressed with a sudden surge of sugar and fat. People who eat large meals must process and store twice as much fat and sugar as those who eat sparingly. These heavy eaters build up stomachs and intestines that are 40 percent larger than in normal eaters.

Although arthritis and gout have not been directly linked to heavy eating, other degenerative diseases have. Eating large meals is a proven risk factor for heart disease, maturity diabetes, and hypertension and, by suppressing the immune system, for cancer. Since all degenerative diseases have similar roots, it appears extremely likely that heavy eating is also a causative factor in the onset of arthritis.

For example, at Prague University, Czechoslovakia, Dr. Paul Fabry conducted a study of 1,133 men aged 60–64. He found that heart disease was significantly greater among those who ate three or fewer meals a day (30.5 percent had heart attacks) than among those who consumed the same amount spread over five meals or more (only 20 percent had heart attacks).

Research has shown that primitive human populations seldom if ever ate large, heavy meals. Instead, they nibbled small amounts of food at frequent intervals.

Our bodies are simply not adapted to handling the stress of coping with large, heavy meals. When Dr. Grant Gwineup, a professor at the University of California at Irvine, changed meal patterns from three standard-sized meals a day to 10 mini-meals, he found that the reduced stress on digestion significantly reduced risk of heart attack.

The Wizardry of Mini-Meals

Many cardiac rehabilitation centers break each standard-sized meal into three mini-meals and serve a total of nine small meals spread over the day. Records kept at these institutions show that obese people who change to eating mini-meals lose approximately two pounds per week without reducing their calorie intake. In less than three months, their serum cholesterol level has frequently returned to normal. The records also show that while recovering from heart disease through mini-meals, some patients simultaneously recover from both osteo and rheumatoid arthritis, and gout.

To eat the mini-meal way, you take your usual breakfast and divide it into three equal portions. You do the same with your usual lunch and dinner. This provides nine mini-meals which you eat throughout the day at approximately 90 minute intervals.

If you prefer, you can divide your normal daily ration into as few as five mini-meals. Or into any larger number you wish. Of course, you will observe the other rules such as eating only when calm and when hungry, and you must still eat slowly and chew each mouthful thoroughly.

People who work find few problems in dovetailing mini-meals into most job schedules. You can begin with one mini-meals at breakfast time, a second during the mid-morning break, a third at lunchtime, a fourth during the mid-afternoon break, a fifth immediately upon reaching home and the rest spread over the evening. You can easily carry fresh, raw foods to work such as nuts, seeds, fruits, salad vegetables, and whole grain bread.

Eating the mini-meal way virtually guarantees freedom from bloating, gas, or indigestion. The meals are so light that digestion is scarcely noticeable and you are permanently freed from ever feeling loggy or distressingly full. Observations have shown that absorption is far better, and the pulse rate seldom rises when small meals are eaten.

There is also a growing body of evidence to show that allergenic foods eaten the mini-meal way are less likely to set off the immune response.

No one with arthritis should fail to change over to the mini-meal way of eating.

Rule #2: Eat Only When Hungry

Much of our eating is done for entertainment or amusement, as a social habit, to relieve boredom or as a stimulant. From now on, eat only when you are actually hungry. If you are not actually hungry, skip a meal.

Rule #3: Eat Only When You Feel Calm and Serene and When the Atmosphere is Peaceful and Relaxed

Never eat when you are tired, tense, sick, upset, or late at night.

If you feel hungry or emotionally tense at the same time, use this quick-relaxation technique. Stand upright and tense all the muscles in your body simultaneously. Hold for eight seconds. Then release. Tense your arms, legs, hands, feet, abdomen, back, neck, and face muscles. If you can't tense them all at once, tense both arms and hands first, hold to the slow count of eight, and release. Then repeat with both legs, with the shoulders and back, with the abdomen and buttocks, and lastly the neck and face.

Next sit or lie down and take six slow, deep breaths. Inhale for four seconds, hold the breath for four seconds, and exhale for four seconds. Take six of these slow, deep inhalations. Then relax and visualize yourself running along a beach with your spine and joints as flexible as a kitten's and with all your arthritis already gone. Keep visualizing yourself as already recovered from arthritis.

By the time your mind tires of this exercise, you will be completely calm and serene and ready to eat.

Rule #4: Eat Slowly and Chew Foods Well

Never eat on the run or against the clock or when in a hurry or while standing up. These are almost certain ways to develop indigestion. A good way to slow down your eating is to use chopsticks

Digestion of all starches and other complex carbohydrates begins in the mouth. The food must be thoroughly chewed so it's broken into smaller pieces and mixed with enzyme-rich saliva. Swallow each mouthful only when it is chewed into a liquid pulp.

Failing to thoroughly chew beans is the reason why many people complain that these foods cause flatulence. (If you still find that beans are gassy, try cooking them together with brown rice and make sure the beans you buy are fresh.)

You will also lose weight faster by eating slowly and chewing more. This is because after eating it takes about ten minutes for a feeling of fullness to register in the brain. By eating more slowly you will feel full before you have eaten as much food.

Rule #5: When to Avoid Liquids with Meals

For people with optimal digestion, drinking fluids with meals isn't a problem. However, if your stomach acid is low and causing you trouble (remember one-third or more of those with rheumatoid arthritis have been found to be lacking in stomach acid), drink little or nothing with meals. Traditional natural health thought says that too much liquid with meals dilutes stomach acid and digestive enzymes thus inhibiting the digestive process.

If you want to try this, don't drink within 20 minutes of eating a standard-sized meal nor for 90 minutes afterwards. With mini-meals, avoid drinking for 10 minutes before eating and for 30 minutes after finishing.

One exception to this rule is pineapple or papaya juice. Both tropical fruits contain protein-digesting enzymes and can be sipped alongside a meal as digestive aids. You can also try drinking a glass of pure water spiked with freshly squeezed lemon juice, an old-time tonic for enhancing gastric and salivary juices and arousing the appetite.

Rule #6: Eat Sparingly but Enjoy It

Several studies on longevity have all found that people who eat sparingly live longer and enjoy better health. As we have already learned, people with optimum health are less prone to arthritis.

Here are several simple techniques that will almost ensure you eat sparingly.

- Before beginning any meal, remove one-fifth of the food from your plate. Then try to leave some food on your plate when you finish.
- After a meal is served, sit and wait a full minute before starting to eat.
- Put down the utensils between each mouthful until food is completely chewed and swallowed. Or if eating with your hands, put your food back on the plate after each bite.
- Bite off or take only a half a mouthful at a time instead of a full mouthful.
- If you are right-handed, eat with the left hand. Or vice versa. This will slow down your eating.
- Keep the refrigerator almost empty.
- Always leave the table feeling slightly hungry (You will fill up naturally in 10–20 minutes as your brain registers that you've eaten enough.)

June R. Loses Her Arthritis by Eating Naturally

When June R. used several eating techniques simultaneously in a natural approach to healing arthritis, she achieved dynamic results.

"I had osteoarthritis and my problem was fifty pounds of surplus fat," June reported while relaxing on the patio of her Arizona retirement home. "This was when I worked in an ad agency and my busy schedule left no time for cleansing or fasting. I had never been able to stick with any diet. Finally, I signed up with a weight-loss clinic that specialized in behavior motivation.

"I was instructed to eat a low-fat, high-fiber diet of fresh natural foods, and I had to prepare it in the 65-20-15 way. Well, I was allowed to eat as much as I wanted provided I ate in the form of nine small meals each spaced ninety minutes apart. I could eat only when I felt hungry and I was to chew each mouthful thoroughly before swallowing. I also agreed to eat only when I felt emotionally calm and relaxed."

All of June's previous diets had stressed low carbohydrate consumption and had left her feeling hungry and tired. This time it was different. She found her complex carbohydrate diet so filling that she actually had to skip two mini-meals each day.

"I never felt hungry and I ate all I wanted," June said. "But I still lost a steady five pounds a week. This natural approach was a powerful system. Without ever counting calories or feeling hungry, in three months my weight dropped right back to normal.

"With every pound I lost, my knees felt better, By the time I was back in a size twelve dress, I was able to walk without any pain and I could even dance.

"I've stayed faithfully with the natural foods diet and the mini-meals, and I've never changed the 65-20-15 formula. All that super-nutrition gradually restored health to my knees. Right now at sixty-five, I'm as flexible and agile as when I was twenty-one. My weight is exactly what it was then. And I don't have a trace of arthritis."

Chapter *17*

Fibromyalgia: An Up and Coming Arthritis

Last but not least we present a separate chapter on fibromyalgia, the incurable arthritis. Or is it?

Not surprising, many of the same nutritional techniques that help osteo and rheumatoid arthritis benefit fibromyalgia. Replacing health-destructive stressor foods with health-rekindling restorative foods is just the first step. Ferreting out allergy foods and implementing the digestive diet plan are also useful.

But there's more. And that's why we've saved fibromyalgia until now. There's still much we don't know about this disease. Doctors have less experience treating fibromyalgia than they do arthritis, but the puzzle pieces are starting to come together.

Before we reveal what natural medicine has to offer for this painful and frustrating condition, a little background on this up and coming arthritis.

 A Waste Basket Diagnosis

Fifteen years ago fibromyalgia, then called fibrositis, was lumped together with other ambiguous and mystifying muscle aches. Since then this up and coming arthritis has grown in leaps and bounds to the point where anywhere from four to six million

277

Americans are afflicted and researchers are scrambling to explain its cause.

One doctor explains this apparent epidemic by describing fibromyalgia as a "waste basket diagnosis," an easy disease into which physicians can toss vague aches and pains of muscles and joints. Increasing stress and poor diets, so typical of modern lives, may be driving fibromyalgia's numbers up.

"Fibromyalgia's symptoms are so vague and difficult to treat, that for a long time doctors denied it existed," are the words of another physician who specializes in this condition. Fibromyalgia's many and varied symptoms don't fit well into any conventional medical diagnostic mold. Yet patients are still complaining.

Elusive and widespread pain and isolated tender points target the almost 700 muscles in a fibromyalgia patient's body. The pain is so exquisite for some that even a simple touch is agony. These individuals are often tired, stiff, anxious, or depressed and have trouble sleeping. The typical fibromyalgia sufferer is a middle-aged woman.

NSAID drugs, standard arthritis medications, don't make most fibromyalgia patients feel better. The usual course of treatment is stress management, exercise as tolerated, psychological counseling, physical therapies like massage, and antidepressants. Antidepressants and muscle relaxants don't solve the problem, but may decrease symptoms. Unfortunately, side effects are a nuisance and after six months or so some of these medicines lose their effectiveness[91].

Is Natural Medicine the Answer?

For the very reason that fibromyalgia doesn't fit into a neat and tidy diagnostic box, may be why this ailment is a prime candidate for natural therapies including nutrition. Because natural medicine takes into account everything about a person—his emotional, mental and physical state, eating patterns, social interactions and lifestyle habits—and digs around for the root cause, natural medicine is better equipped to handle unruly diseases like fibromyalgia. There's other reasons, too.

The emotional and physical demands of modern day life have been implicated in triggering or aggravating fibromyalgia. The stress of constant loud noise, too little sleep, pollutants, chemicals and drugs, overwork, and emotional trauma are problems. Again, natural practitioners are experts at addressing these concerns.

Fibromyalgia has been compared to chronic fatigue syndrome, multiple allergy syndrome, multiple chemical sensitivity, and immune dysfunction, conditions commonly diagnosed and treated by natural health practitioners. Many of these illnesses also improve when food choices improve.

It's interesting, too, that fibromyalgia may be autoimmune in nature and can occur alongside rheumatoid arthritis, lupus, and other types of arthritis[92]. If this is so, then the very same nutritional strategies we've suggested for arthritis should help.

Indigestion Might Make Your Muscles Hurt

The idea that diet causes muscle pain is an old one. The old fashioned term "allergic toxemia" describing vague muscle aches and pains, fatigue, weakness, headaches, and sleeplessness sounds very much like fibromyalgia. The solution is to avoid allergens and toxic chemicals—no different from our arthritis plan.

Further evidence linking fibromyalgia to digestion was found at Beaumont Hospital in Dublin, Ireland. Doctors discovered that 70 percent of their fibromyalgia patients had irritable bowel syndrome (IBS), a large intestine disorder where constipation alternates with diarrhea, and gas, nausea, abdominal pain, loss of appetite, and depression or anxiety are present. Not surprisingly 65 percent of their IBS patients had fibromyalgia[93]. Is there connection between these two afflictions? Possibly, say these Irish researchers.

Irritable bowel syndrome is treated much like other gut disorders. Fiber rich foods are stressed, food allergies are hunted down, and yogurt or lactobacillus supplementation is used when gut flora is out of balance. Peppermint oil or tea calms down bowel irritability.

Dr. Donovan from Bastyr University recalls a particular fibromyalgia patient whom, after seeing another natural health specialist, improved 50 percent. Still, she felt there was more that could be done to decrease her pain. She visited Dr. Donovan who investigated her digestive function and checked for leaky gut syndrome. Sure enough, there was a problem. He put her on his digestive diet plan (similar to the one described in Chapter 6) plus some other individualized therapies. Within a few months, her muscle pain was nearly gone.

Is Fibromyalgia an Allergic Reaction or a Chemical Sensitivity?

Eliminating offending foods helps a broad assortment of body-wide complaints including fibromyalgia-like symptoms—muscle pain, headache, sleep disturbance, irritability, rapid heart rate, and bowel troubles[94]. Widespread allergies are also associated with chronic fatigue syndrome, a condition that is often compared to fibromyalgia[92].

Ten middle-aged fibromyalgia patients were placed on a three-week regimen of vegetarian meals and fasting by doctors from the Department of Preventive Medicine at the University of Oslo in Norway. This cleansing program cleared these subjects' bloodstream's of many free radicals, those same pesky molecules that aggravate arthritis in general[95].

Muscular pain is one symptom of environmental illness, a devastating affliction where any number of foods and chemicals, ranging from perfume to household cleaners, are intolerable. Isn't it strange, then, that fibromyalgia can also be triggered by toxic compounds like chemotherapeutic drugs, silicone breast implants[92], or phenobarbital, an antiseizure medicine? Even vitamin A, a normally benign and vital substance, can create aching muscles in exceedingly high dosages[96].

It therefore makes sense that once you've solved any digestive dilemmas, use the same suggestions offered in Chapters 7, 8, and 9 to track down allergy foods, and toss them from your diet. Keep chemical exposure to a minimum, and treat your liver—the extraordinary toxin-filtering organ well.

One Doctor's Theory Clearly Explains Fibromyalgia

While most doctors are baffled by fibromyalgia's elusive nature, Dr. Jorge D. Flechas, a family practice physician from Hendersonville, North Carolina, has found the answer. Claiming an 80 percent cure rate, Dr. Flechas' hours of research, reasoning, and working with 600 patients with fibromyalgia have rewarded him with the following hypothesis.

"Fibromyalgia is basically a lack of energy probably due to an inherited bad set of mitochondria," explains Dr. Flechas. Energy for the entire body is produced by mitochondria, small power packs that reside within each cell. Mitochondria make energy by converting raw oxygen and nutrients into adenosine triphosphate (ATP), the high-energy compound that powers most functions in your body.

People with fibromyalgia tend to be low in ATP (98) and hence stamina. This condition also runs in families.

Fibromyalgia shows up more in older people whose hormone levels are dropping. Most significant is when the adrenal hormone dehydroepiandosterone (DHEA) falls. DHEA is the "mother" hormone from which other hormones can be made. Not only that, but DHEA is intricately involved in mitochondrial ATP-energy production—often malfunctioning in those with fibromyalgia.

It's also possible, says Dr. Flechas, that oxytocin, best known as the breastfeeding hormone, is low in those with fibromyalgia. This supposedly female-only hormone is actually present in both men and women. Although scientifically established, few physicians recognize oxytocin's extensive role in relieving pain, keeping the mind sharp, counteracting anxiety and depression, and controlling circulation. All these functions are compromised in fibromyalgia.

One Doctor's Prescription for Fibromyalgia

One of the first tests Jorge Flechas, MD performs on his fibromyalgia patients is the DHEA-sulfate blood test. If levels are low, he prescribes DHEA replacement therapy. Patients continue with this treatment until their DHEA reservoirs equal those of a normal 30 year old. Dr. Flechas keeps his fibromyalgia patients on a maintenance dose of this hormone medication for life.

(By the way, research points to DHEA as an effective medication for other types of arthritis too such as lupus[99] and rheumatoid arthritis[100]. Ask your doctor.)

A British research team found estrogen replacement therapy worked well in alleviating fibromyalgia symptoms in menopausal women[101]. However, because the body can use DHEA to make its own estrogen, supplementing with this adrenal hormone helps just as well.

Oxytocin is another hormone Dr. Flechas supplements in his patients with fibromyalgia. There is no laboratory test currently available to judge oxytocin levels. However, this North Carolina physician finds that most of his fibromyalgia patients benefit from oxytocin therapy.

Obviously these therapies can only be implemented with your doctor's cooperation. We include them so you may explore these options with your physician.

Taking the "P" Out of Pain

Studies reveal that substance P, the pain sensitive neurotransmitter, is four times higher in the cerebrospinal fluid of fibromyalgia patients when compared to healthy individuals[92]. This may explain why those with fibromyalgia complain about having a very low threshold of pain, and why they hurt in general.

Luckily nature serves up many food-medicines that soak up substance P and reduce pain. In 1992, K. C. Srivastava and T. Mustafa from Denmark discovered that all 10 of their patients with muscular discomfort who used powdered ginger got better[80]. Fibromyalgia wasn't specified as the cause of achy muscles in Srivastava's study, but it stands to reason that spicing your food with ginger (and substance P-depleting cayenne pepper) may help.

Relaxing Muscles with Magnesium

At the Central Hospital of Toulon in France, J. Eisinger and associates found magnesium levels in fibromyalgia patients to be on the low side[102]. Magnesium is another key participant in the mitochondrial energy cycle. This mineral also relaxes tense muscles and assists with sleep—both problematic for the fibromyalgic sufferer.

Magnesium is housed mainly in whole grains, dark-green vegetables, and nuts, foods ignored in the average American dinner. Doctors who treat fibromyalgia find magnesium capsules useful, too.

Using Fruits and Vegetables to Cure Aching Muscles

If you need one more reason why you should eat all your fruits and vegetables, here it is. Oxytocin relies on inositol, abundantly found in vegetables, fruits, nuts, legumes, and whole grains like brown rice, to interact with cells and participate in other bodily functions. Without inositol, myoinositol or "muscle sugar" drops.

When Dr. Flechas traveled to Mexico, where rice is a staple food, he was astonished by how few people complained of fibromyalgia. Besides shunning vegetables and fruits, most Americans turn to potatoes or bread instead of rice as their favorite starchy entree.

Malic acid is the other missing ingredient in standard western fare. Found in apples and other tart fruits, malic acid is another important member of the energy cycle occurring inside the mitochondria. DHEA adrenal production is stimulated by malic acid too. People who neglect fresh fruit are missing energy-dependent malic acid, and may be shortchanging themselves on vital DHEA.

But it's not just fruits and vegetables that are absent from our lives. It's the realization, as illustrated by the dozens of stories in this book, that we have a fountain of health and youth already within each of us. Through harmful habits of eating and living, we turn the fountain off. Yet we can always turn the fountain on again by replacing our health-destroying eating and living habits with beneficial health-restoring foods and by cultivating other habits designed to produce high-level wellness.

That is the message of the natural approach to healing described in this book. Through learning all about arthritis and all the medical options and alternatives available—not merely conventional ones—we can each become a medically educated layperson thoroughly capable of taking control of our own health and taking an active role in our own recovery.

No drug, injection, or surgery can tap our wellsprings of inner health. Only you can turn on the recuperative and rejuvenating powers that live within.

In the final analysis, overcoming arthritis—or even fibromyalgia—is something that begins with you making a decision to get well. If you need help along the way, turn to one of the many natural medical practitioners, ready and willing to help you turn on your fountain of health.

Dictionary of

Restorative Foods

We suggest tossing out stressor foods to improve your arthritis and replacing them with natural restorative foods. But did you know food can be your medicine too? Unlike conventional drugs, that work hard and fast sometimes jolting your body so much that the side effects are unsettling, food-medicines heal with a quiet and gentle hand.

The line between plant-herbs (from which many drugs originate) and plant-foods is sometimes a hazy one. The continuum runs from purely edible plants to mild food-medicines to plant-foods with moderate healing properties to potentially toxic herbs.

The restorative foods described below are foods the body needs to supply the energy, minerals, vitamins, chlorophyll, enzymes, and protein required in the healing process. Some of these foods also have medicinal qualities. This concept of food-medicines explains why primitive cultures, who eat a variety of whole, fresh, raw, and often wild plants, avoid many modern day ailments like arthritis.

Another basic law of natural healing is that given half a chance the body will heal itself. While medicinal foods encourage this process along, healing is a biological operation that can be accomplished only by the body's own recuperative and rejuvenative powers. When the cause of disease is removed, the body becomes a self-healing entity provided it is supplied with the biological necessities. These include pure air and water, rest, emotional calm, and natural, nutrient-rich foods.

To ensure that the body assimilates and utilizes these restorative foods—thereby maximizing the healing process—they should ideally be eaten in proper combinations. This is particularly important for anyone with digestive disturbances. You may not find food combining necessary if your gastrointestinal tract is functioning at full efficiency. The basic rules for proper food combining are outlined in Chapter 12. If, however, you experience any gas, flatulence or other form of indigestion after eating certain combinations of vegetables, fruits, or other foods, you can probably avoid it in the future by observing the following, more detailed rules for successful food combining.

Protein foods combine well with green vegetables and with acid fruits, but not with starches or sweet fruits.

Starchy vegetables combine well with other starches including most cereals.

Green vegetables combine well with vegetables, proteins, and starches but not with most fruits.

Cereals, mostly grains, combine well with most green and starchy vegetables and with fats. They are not always compatible with fruits, especially acid fruits. However, most sub-acid and sweet fruits may be safely mixed with most breakfast cereals.

Acid fruits combine reasonably well with sub-acid fruits and with protein but should not be mixed with starches.

Sub-acid fruits combine reasonably well with acid fruits and may be mixed in reasonable amounts with breakfast cereals or dairy foods.

Sweet fruits combine well with sub-acid fruits but not with acid fruits. They do not mix well with proteins.

Neutral fruits mix well with sub-acid fruits and with green vegetables.

Most of the restorative foods in the following list are identified by food class so that you may combine them properly. All foods of the same type are compatible and may be safely mixed and eaten together. (*Example*: broccoli, Brussels sprouts, cabbage, cauliflower, celery, chard, chives, collards, and cucumber are all classified as green vegetables and can be safely eaten together at the same meal.)

Most natural foods also belong to food families based on their origin. For example, most melons, pumpkins, cucumbers, and squash are descendants of the gourd and belong to the gourd family. Since all foods belonging to any one family are genetically similar, when a person develops an allergy to one food they may be allergic to other foods of the same family.

The significance of food families in tracking down allergies is described in Chapter 8. To assist you in identifying other members of any food family to which you may be allergic, the family to which each food belongs is (where known) listed below.

While all foods which follow are nutritionally helpful to the body in recovering from arthritic disease, you should not eat any to which you know you are allergic or sensitive.

Know too, that this list is by no means complete. We've mentioned most of the healing foods described in our book, but there are numerous other restorative foods out there waiting for you to discover. Be adventurous in your quest for health and by all means try other restorative foods available to you.

Acerola (*Barbados Cherry*). This red-fluted cherry grows on hedges and bushes in South Florida. It is delicious when eaten raw. Since the acerola is a phenomenally rich source of vitamin C, it is of great value in helping the body overcome the aching and swelling of arthritic joints. (A close relative is the pitanga or Surinam cherry.) Class: *acid fruit*.

Alfalfa: (see Beans)

Almond: plum family. Fresh, whole, shelled, unsalted almonds are rich in protein and are a good source of potassium, magnesium, calcium, essential fatty acids, and phosphorus. Almonds go well with vegetable salads or with citrus. You can also try almond milk. Class: *protein*.

Amaranth: grass family. This energizing non-gluten grain was originally a staple of the Aztecs. Small amaranth seeds range from light yellow in color to purplish black and are packed with protein, lysine, calcium, and phosphorus, and low in calories. Amaranth leaves can also be eaten; amaranth flour is useful in baking. Class: *cereal*.

Apple: apple family. Eating unpeeled, apples aids the body in healing arthritis by supplying essential pepsin, and malic acid for those with fibromyalgia. When fresh apples are unavailable, dried apples may be eaten; they are also a good substitute candy. Apple cider vinegar appears to benefit the digestive system and fresh apple juice makes a pleasant drink. However, most nutrients in apple butter and apple jelly have been lost through processing. Class: *sub-acid fruit*.

Apricot: plum family. This delicious fruit is rich in iron and other minerals. Dried apricots are acceptable if free of preservatives like sulphur dioxide. Instead of cooking dried apricots, soften them in water overnight. Class: *sub-acid fruit* (sweet fruit when dried).

Artichoke: aster family. The several varieties of this tuber, including the French and Jerusalem artichoke, are good sources of potassium, iron, magnesium, and calcium as well as vitamins A and C and B-complex. The Jerusalem artichoke also supplies the "friendly" bugs of your GI tract with food called fracto-oligo saccharides. (Garlic, onions, and asparagus have FOS, too.) Artichokes can be eaten raw or briefly baked or steamed. Class: *starchy vegetable*.

Asparagus: lily family. These succulent shoots supply nutrients which the body uses in purifying cells and kidneys, an essential step in overall recovery from arthritis. Asparagus shoots may be eaten raw or lightly steamed for a few minutes, after which they should be eaten promptly before they become limp and lose taste. Class: *green vegetable*.

Avocado: laurel family. This versatile food, available in different varieties through much of the year, combines well with both fruits and vegetables. It is ripe when slightly soft and may be mixed into fruit or vegetable salads, used as a spread on celery sticks or on whole grain bread or made into guacamole. The avocado supplies healthy monounsaturated fats and is rich in essential nutrients needed by the body during recovery from arthritis. Class: *neutral fruit*.

Bamboo shoots: grass family. Bamboo shoot tips are obtainable from most grocery stores. They are valued by Chinese and Japanese as an aid to the body in expelling toxins and in helping lower blood pressure. They may be eaten raw or cooked for a few minutes. Class: *starchy vegetable*.

Banana: banana family. Bananas are one of the best sources of potassium, a nutrient essential to the body during the healing process. Bananas speckled with brown dots are the most ripe and sweet; partly green ones are often starchy and may not ripen fully. Besides being used in fruit salads or eaten on bread, bananas may be frozen to form a natural ice cream. A larger variety with angular sides, the plantain, is often baked. Class: *sweet fruit*.

Barley: grass family. Only unpearled (unrefined) barley should be eaten. It can be cooked as a breakfast cereal (one cup of barley to four cups of water) with raisins added while cooking. Barley is a good source of energy and B vitamins. Class: *cereal*.

Beans: legume family. The best way to eat beans is to sprout them. Otherwise, they should be cooked in a pressure cooker or crockpot. Approximately 20 percent of dried beans is protein. Soybeans are an important source of iron, potassium, unsaturated fatty acids, and healing saponins. An exceedingly diverse bean, soy is available as soy milk, soy cheese or yogurt, soy ice cream, tofu, tempeh, miso (soy paste), soy flour and soynuts. Butter and lima beans also abound with vitamins and minerals, especially iron. Mung beans, used for sprouting, supply a wide assortment of vitamins and minerals which are often deficient in persons suffering from arthritis. String beans are also rich in calcium, magnesium, and potassium. *Alfalfa*, an important food in arthritis recovery, is also a legume. Class: *protein*.

Beechnut: beech family. This small northern nut is high in vegetable protein, unsaturated fatty acids, and energy. Class: *protein*.

Beets: goosefoot family. Beets are best eaten raw after being grated and sprinkled on vegetable salads. They may also be lightly steamed, baked, or made into a soup. The nutritional value of cooked beets may be enhanced by lightly steaming the beet greens, which are rich in iron and other vital minerals, and eating them with the beets. Either raw, or cooked with greens, beets supply important nutrients used by the body in recovery from arthritis by supporting the liver. Class: *starchy vegetable*.

Blackberry: rose family. Nutrients in this berry, which grows on wild or cultivated brambles in cool, northern areas, are utilized by the body in purifying the bloodstream and digestive tract during recovery from arthritic disease. Their high proanthocyanidin content, the black, blue, and red pigment in these and other fruits, helps heal weakened joints and other tissues. Blueberries and loganberries have similar nutritional qualities. These berries should be eaten raw; they are delicious with breakfast cereals. Class: *sub-acid fruits*.

Brazil nut: sapucaia family. This South American import is high in calcium, phosphorous, iron, vegetable protein, calories, and unsaturated fat. Class: *protein*.

Broccoli: cruciferous family. When the raw small green heads are chopped up in a salad they supply nutrients which aid the body in cleaning out harmful free radicals. Alternatively, broccoli may be split and lightly steamed. Class: *green vegetable*.

Brussels sprouts: cruciferous family. Sprouts taste best when about an inch in diameter. Chop and mix them in a raw vegetable salad; or steam for 8–10 minutes. They supply nutrients which aid the body in repairing distressed joints. Class: *green vegetable*.

Buckwheat: rhubarb family. While usually grouped with grains, this is a fruit (and in no way related to wheat). Its robust flavor and nutritious assortment of calcium, lysine, vitamin E, and B-vitamins make it a good cold weather food. It is considered medicinal for the kidneys. Kasha is the hulled version of buckwheat; unhulled or whole buckwheat is only suitable for sprouting. You can also eat buckwheat as flour (good in pancakes) or soba, a Japanese buckwheat pasta. Class: *cereal*.

Cabbage: cruciferous family. The numerous varieties of early and late, green and purple cabbage are good sources of iron, calcium, and other nutrients used by the body in expelling toxins during recovery from arthritis. Cabbage is delicious when raw, especially the purple type. The outer leaves are richest in calcium, so don't discard them. Cabbage may also be cooked lightly till crisp but never, as many restaurants do, till soggy. Class: *green vegetable*.

Cactus fruit: tuna family. Widely available in the Southwest and Mexico, where it is called the tuna or prickly pear, cactus fruit is a tasty, natural food. It must be peeled before eating. Class: *sub-acid fruit*.

Canistel (eggfruit). This soft, yellow tropical fruit is fairly common in South Florida and is a valuable source of vitamin C. Class: *sweet fruit*.

Canola: cabbage family. Canola is the Canadian name for rapeseed (a name that never caught on in North America), originally popular in Europe and India. The nutty, brownish canola seed can be added to foods, or more likely canola oil with its inflammation-fighting monounsaturated fats may be added to salads and other foods. Class: *protein*.

Carambola. This oval, five-sided tropical fruit is often seen in South Florida. It is rich in vitamins and minerals utilized by the body for purifying and healing. Class: *acid fruit*.

Carob: legume family. The pods of the carob tree may be eaten as fruit. More commonly, they are ground into carob powder and sold in health food stores for making a healthful beverage or as a chocolate substitute. Carob powder is a good source of vitamin A and the

B-complex plus calcium, iron, copper, and magnesium. Be sure any carob you buy is sugar-free. Class: *sweet fruit*.

Carrot: parsley family. Eaten raw, carrots supply the body with vitamin A and other nutrients which are utilized in restoring balance to the immune system and endocrine glands. Small, young carrots are best for eating raw, they may be eaten whole or grated, sliced or shredded. Larger, older carrots may be steamed, mashed, or made into a soup or juice. Class: *starchy vegetable*.

Cashew nut: cashew family. This desirable nut is sold shelled because an acid in the shell can blister flesh. In shelling, the nuts are twice heated to 350°F hence they are more liable to turn rancid than most other nuts. Class: *protein*.

Cauliflower: cruciferous family. Best chopped up fine while raw and added to a vegetable salad, cauliflower contains nutrients utilized by the body for restoring carbohydrate metabolism. Older people, who may find difficulty digesting cauliflower raw, may steam it briefly. Class: *green vegetable*.

Cayenne Pepper: (see Pepper)

Celery: parsley family. Eaten whole along with the leaves or chopped in a salad, raw celery is a good source of calcium and other important nutrients utilized by the body during recovery from arthritis and other degenerative diseases. Celery seeds are a fine diuretic, good for arthritic swelling. Class: *green vegetable*.

Chard: goosefoot family. Chard leaves are high in potassium, calcium, iron, and vitamin A and when eaten raw supply the body with nutrients utilized during arthritis recovery. Class: *green vegetable*.

Cherry: plum family. Raw cherries supply iron, magnesium, and other nutrients required by the body while restoring health following arthritis or other degenerative diseases. The darker the cherries, the richer they are in iron, magnesium, and antioxidant flavonoids. Cherries in pies and preserves have lost much of their nutritional value. Class: *sub-acid fruit*.

Chestnut: beech family. A good source of iron and phosphorus, chestnuts are difficult to digest raw owing to their tannic acid content. Lightly roasted, they make a delicious addition to vegetable salads or to chicken or turkey served with sweet potatoes. Class: *protein*.

Chicken: quail family. Chicken eaten without the skin is a desirable low fat source of whole protein and is also high in phosphorus and potassium. Class: *protein*.

Chives: lily family. The slender leaves of this onion plant can be chopped fine and used to flavor salads and soups. Class: *green vegetable*.

Citrus: citrus family. All members of the citrus family—oranges, grapefruit, lemons, limes, tangerines, and tangelos—are good sources of vitamin C while the white outer pith contains bioflavonoids which help keep the arteries flexible. Citrus supplies the body with nutrients for healing arthritic joints. Drinking fresh juice is slightly less desirable than eating the fruit. However, the juice of limes or lemons makes a tasty addition to herb teas, vegetable and fruit salads, and over tropical fruits. Class: *acid fruit*.

Coconut: palm family. This large nut is a good source of protein but is high in saturated fat. Coconut, if eaten, should be whole and fresh. Drain out the water and drink it. Green coconuts sold in Florida have meat that is so soft, it can be eaten with a spoon. Older, harder coconut meat can be cut up and eaten like other nuts or grated and sprinkled on vegetable salads. Class: *protein*.

Cod: cod family. A superior source of low-fat protein, this valuable food fish also supplies phosphorus and potassium. Highly recommended. Class: *protein*.

Collards: cruciferous family. This headless cabbage is an important source of calcium and other nutrients required by the body for healing arthritis. The leaves can be eaten raw in a salad or lightly steamed for a few minutes. Class: *green vegetable*.

Corn: grass family. Eaten raw when young or briefly steamed when mature, corn is a valuable body-building staple. The fact that it is classified as a vegetable when young and fresh, and as a starchy cereal when older and dried indicates that young, fresh corn eaten raw is less likely to be allergenic. Unfortunately, corn products such as corn syrup, meal, or starch are denatured by heat during manufacture while hominy, another form of corn, may be contaminated by chemicals used in removing its outer shell. Class: *vegetable* when fresh and young; *cereal* when older and dried.

Cottage cheese: bovid family. Non-fat cottage cheese is a superior source of whole protein and a good source of calcium, vitamins B_6

and B_{12}, phosphorus, and riboflavin. It makes a splendid salad dressing and also blends well with sub-acid fruits. Class: *protein*.

Cranberry: heath family. Too tart and acidic to eat raw, the cranberry must be lightly cooked. Because large amounts of sugar are added to commercially prepared cranberries, home preparation is recommended. Even cooked, the cranberry is a valuable source of essential nutrients used by the body in recovering from gout. Class: *acid fruit*.

Cucumber: gourd family. High in potassium and other minerals, this watery vegetable is a mild diuretic. A mixture of fresh cucumber and carrot juice aids the body in purifying itself of uric acid. Pickled cucumbers are nutritionally valueless. Try, also, to buy cucumbers that have not had their skins oiled by the supermarket. Class: *green vegetable*.

Currant: gooseberry family. Of the three varieties of currant—red, black, and white—the red is richest in minerals. Currants mixed with freshly grated coconut and rolled into balls make a fine natural candy. Class: *acid fruit*.

Dandelion: aster family. The small, young leaves of cultivated varieties like the Improved Broad Leaf are a welcome addition to salads. Wild dandelions are bitter but helpful for digestion. Dandelions can also be cooked like spinach. Raw dandelions, or dandelion root and leaf tea, contain nutrients valuable to the body in restoring health and cleansing the liver. Class: *green vegetable*.

Date: palm family. A good source of iron and potassium, dates are an excellent substitute for candy. They should be eaten in limited amounts because they are high in fruit sugar. Class: *sweet fruit*.

Dulse: This American salt water algae is an important source of iron, calcium, iodine, and phosphorus. The dried, purple leaves are sold in most health food stores and they impart a zesty tang when chopped and sprinkled on salads or other foods. The leaves may also be chewed alone and are nutritionally superior to the powdered or tablet form of dulse.

Eggplant: nightshade family. Baked together with tomatoes and garlic, this purple vegetable provides a tasty dish. It contains nutrients used by the body to restore sound digestion. Class: *green vegetable*.

Endives: aster family. The broad leafed variety of endive is also known as escarole. Endive should be chopped and mixed into a green salad since it is rather bitter when eaten alone. A good source of potassium, calcium, and phosphorus, it supplies essential nutrients utilized by the body in promoting digestion. Class: *green vegetable*.

Figs: mulberry family. Their high iron and mineral content make figs nutritionally valuable to the body in its efforts to cleanse the bowels and restore sound digestion. Fresh figs are preferable. Dried figs make a good substitute for candy but should be eaten only in limited quantities due to their high sugar content. Class: *sweet fruit*.

Filbert: beech family. Known also as the hazelnut or cobnut, the filbert has a high content of calcium and phosphorus and is a good source of healthful fats and protein. Class: *protein*.

Flax seeds: Also known as linseed, these omega-6 rich seeds are typically used to regulate bowels. They can be sprinkled on food or ground up to create a mushy meal. Flax seed oil helps decrease pain and inflammation in joints. Psyllium seeds have medicinal qualities similar to flax seeds, but comes from a different plant. Class: *protein*.

Garlic: lily family. The cloves of this hardy bulb supply essential nutrients used by the body in fighting infections and in restoring balance to immunity and digestive systems. Add chopped cloves to stews and steamed dishes or rub them over a wooden salad bowl before filling. Stores also sell squeezers for extracting the juice from garlic cloves that can be dripped into almost any kind of cooked food. Garlic oil is also available in capsules. Class: *vegetable*.

Ginger: This major spice and food flavoring agent also possesses numerous medicinal properties. Add the chopped up root to sautéed vegetables or fish, or drink ginger root tea to ease digestion and reduce inflammation. Powdered ginger is less medicinal than the fresh root. Class: *vegetable*.

Gooseberry: gooseberry family. Eaten raw, this delicious northern berry supplies nutrients valuable to the body during arthritis recovery. Class: *acid fruit*.

Grape: grape family. Valued for nutrients used by the body in excreting uric acid, raw, fresh grapes are delicious when eaten alone or in a fruit salad. Raisins, which are dried grapes, have a high mineral content, are equally desirable and may be added to many foods to impart added flavor. Fresh grape juice is a commendable beverage. Class: *sub-acid fruit.*

Guava: myrtle family. The apple of the tropics, the guava grows wild in South Florida. Although the guava is used in jams, jellies, and paste, it is best when eaten raw; simply peel it and munch. The guava contains nutrients utilized by the body in restoring health to the circulatory system. Class: *sub-acid fruit.*

Haddock: cod family. A filet of this deep ocean fish supplies 18.3 grams of whole protein yet only .1 grams of fat. The haddock is also a dependable source of calcium, potassium, phosphorus, and magnesium. Class: *protein.*

Herring: Economical as well as nutritious, herring is high in both protein and pain-relieving omega-3 oils. Their high fat content makes herring more perishable. Fresh and dried versions are more desirable than pickled or smoked. Class: *protein.*

Kale: cruciferous family. The curled, wrinkled leaves of this headless cabbage are rich in nutrients utilized by the body during recovery from arthritis. Kale is best eaten raw in salads, or it may be lightly steamed. Class: *green vegetable.*

Kelp: This seaweed is an important source of iron, calcium, phosphorus, and iodine as well as vegetable protein. It is usually eaten as a zesty seasoning sprinkled on salads and other foods.

Kohlrabi: cruciferous family. When peeled, this white, nutty vegetable may be eaten raw or chopped up in salads, or lightly steamed or baked. It is reputed to contain nutrients valuable to the body in restoring health to the urinary system. Class: *starchy vegetable.*

Lettuce: aster family. A good source of calcium, iron, potassium and phosphorus, the green outer leaves of lettuce are also rich in chlorophyll. All are essential for arthritis recovery and for maintaining health afterwards. Loose-leafed lettuce, such as Romaine and Bibb varieties, are nutritionally superior to the tight-packed Iceberg variety. Class: *green vegetable.*

Lychee: Also called the litchi, this nut-like fruit grows in Southern California and Florida. Lychees are best eaten fresh but are also available dried, when they taste like raisins. Fresh lychees are often mixed in with tropical fruits while dried lychees can be soaked and boiled for adding to vegetable casseroles or rice dishes. Class: *sub-acid fruit* (*sweet fruit* when dried).

Mackerel: mackerel family. Another highly desirable fatty fish, the mackerel is available fresh during spring and summer. It is packed with protein too. Class: *protein*.

Mamey: A russet-skinned tropical fruit found in South Florida and Mexico, the mamey has a dark-orange flesh rich in vitamins and minerals utilized by the body in normalizing carbohydrate metabolism. Class: *sub-acid fruit*.

Mango: cashew family. The large, oval varieties of mango now cultivated in South Florida rank among the most delicious and healthful foods in existence. The mango is ripe when slightly soft and when the skin turns yellow-red. Mango, in the form of chutney or preserves has lost most of its nutrients. Class: *sub-acid fruit*.

Melons: gourd family. Their mildly diuretic effect makes melons such as the honeydew or cantaloupe helpful to the body in excreting gout-producing uric acid and other toxins. Chilled watermelon also makes a satisfying substitute for ice cream. Watermelon seeds may be chewed and eaten, or crushed and used to make a healthful herb tea. (Steep one tablespoon of the crushed seeds in a cup of hot water for one hour; then reheat and serve.) If you find that melons do not combine well for you with other fruits, simply eat melons alone. Class: *neutral fruit*.

Millet: grass family. Cooked millet makes a satisfying breakfast cereal, especially when served with fruit. This gluten-free grain may also be used in baking. Class: *cereal*.

Mint: Peppermint, spearmint, and other members of the mint family are relaxing and soothing to the digestion. They can either be drunk as warm teas or add the fresh leaves to main dishes. A dab of peppermint oil rubbed on swollen joints eases pain.

Mushroom: yeast family. Though not always easy to digest raw, this edible fungi is a good source of vitamins and minerals. Try adding it to raw salads. If you have difficulty digesting raw mushrooms, add them to a soup or use them in other cooked dishes. Class: *neutral vegetable*. (See Shiitake mushroom.)

Mustard: cruciferous family. Cultivated mustard greens add zest to a vegetable salad, or they may be lightly steamed. Eaten raw, mustard greens supply chlorophyll and other nutrients essential to the body in recovery from arthritis. Their bitter taste actually enhances digestive secretions. Class: *green vegetable*.

Oats: grass family. This mineral-rich grain is probably the finest choice among breakfast cereals. Serve with *sub-acid* fruits such as apples, pears, peaches, or with melons. Use only the unprocessed oats. Contrary to kitchen folklore, it can be cooked almost as quickly as "quick cooking" finely-chopped oats. Oatbran is another fast cooking healthful cereal. Class: *cereal*.

Okra: mallow family. Okra's mucilaginous content is soothing to the digestive tract, and it can be cooked in a very brief time. Okra is delicious when baked with tomatoes, garlic and onions. Class: *green vegetable*.

Olive: olive family. Due to chemical additives, salt, and processing, pickled olives have little nutritional value. However, cold-pressed olive oil is a fine dressing for salads and other foods, especially when mixed on a one-to-one basis with lemon juice. High in omega-3 fatty acids, this flavorful oil reduces painful joints. Use olive oil only when fresh.

Onion: lily family. Raw chives, leeks, shallots, and scallions enhance the flavor of any vegetable salad. Large yellow, purple, or white onions can be cooked or steamed with other vegetables, or made into an onion casserole. Onions have similar but milder medicinal properties to garlic. Class: *green vegetable*.

Papaya: pawpaw family. This melon-like tropical fruit ranges up to the size of a football. Peel to eat. In the hollow center of the orange-colored meat are scores of black seeds rich in papain, a protein digesting enzyme. Papayas are ripe when the green skin is streaked with yellow. They are a good source of vitamin C and potassium and, when slightly unripe, of papain. The papaya is one of the great tropical fruits. The best are grown in Florida and Mexico, but smaller varieties from Hawaii are carried year round in many supermarkets. The papaya blends well with other sub-acid fruits. Try sprinkling it with lime juice or mix a papaya-pineapple cocktail to drink with meals. Class: *sub-acid fruit*.

Parsley: parsley family. This herb is rich in vitamins and minerals of which many arthritic sufferers are deficient. Chopped parsley should be liberally used to flavor salads and other vegetable foods. Parsley can also be added as a flavoring to vegetable juices. As a juice it is mildly diuretic. Eaten raw, it supplies the body with nutrients utilized for excreting toxins. Class: *green vegetable.*

Pea: legume family. Fresh garden peas, especially edible pod varieties, combine fiber, protein, vitamins, and minerals in a single delicious food. Mix them into vegetable salads or eat them alone as a snack. Dried peas, including lentils, are second choice but are still a good source of vegetable protein. If you must cook peas, do so for as brief a time as possible. Pea or lentil soup containing carrots, rice, celery, onion, potato, tomato, and garlic is a tasty, nutritional meal. Class: *green vegetable.*

Peach: plum family. Peaches and nectarines are easily digested and supply important nutrients that the body requires to recover from arthritis and stay healthy. Peaches blend well with other sub-acid fruits; fresh (not canned) peach halves also taste good with cottage cheese. Dried peaches, if free of preservatives, are rich in minerals; they can be lightly stewed and served as compote. Class: *sub-acid fruit.*

Peanuts: legume family. Actually a bean, the peanut is a good source of energy and protein together with potassium, calcium, phosphorus, iron, and unsaturated fat. Freshly made peanut butter or cold-pressed, unrefined peanut oil retains most of the peanut's nutrients. If not kept refrigerated, both butter and oil will soon turn rancid. Try spreading peanut butter on celery sticks and use as a snack or as refreshments at a party. Class: *protein.*

Pear: apply family. A desirable, low calorie fruit, the pear blends well in fruit salads and may be cut and served on breakfast cereal. Leave the skin on if possible. Dried pears are acceptable only if free of preservatives. Class: *sub-acid fruits.*

Pecan: walnut family. This valued protein food is also a good source of calcium, phosphorous, potassium, and unsaturated fat. It can be eaten with salads or as a snack. Class: *protein.*

Peppers: nightshade family. A rich source of vitamin C when eaten raw, the green pepper enhances the taste of any vegetable salad. It may also be stuffed with cabbage, carrots, and tomatoes and lightly baked. Hot peppers, especially cayenne, are wonderful stomach healing, anti-inflammatory food medicines. If you like hot food, spice your meals up with cayenne and other hot peppers. Class: *green vegetable.*

Persimmon: plum family. This reddish-orange fruit comes in light- and dark-skinned varieties. The dark-fleshed fruit may be eaten before it is actually ripe, but light-fleshed persimmons are astringent until perfectly ripe. Class: *sweet fruit*.

Pine nut: conifer family. Called pinon or pignola nut in its native Southwest, the pine nut is widely available in most health food stores. Although rich in protein, it is easily chewed and goes well with vegetable salads. Since they soon spoil, pine nuts should be kept refrigerated. Class: *protein*.

Pineapple: pineapple family. Imported from Hawaii, Puerto Rico, and Mexico, the pineapple is readily available throughout the year. Its rich juice, fiber, and protein-digesting bromelain enzyme give the pineapple special nutrient values essential to the body in reversing arthritis. Fresh pineapple juice is also a healthful beverage. Canned pineapple or pineapple juice should never be eaten. Fresh pineapple is delicious on breakfast cereal or mixed with papaya. Class: *acid fruit*.

Pistachio nut: cashew family. Unless purchased from health food stores, most pistachio nuts have been denatured by roasting, dyeing, and salting. They are a fine source of protein, unsaturated fat, and energy. Class: *protein*.

Plum: plum family. The numerous varieties of plum are all healthful foods. Prunes are dried plums and are a good natural laxative. Prunes can be soaked overnight and eaten without stewing or boiling. Class: *sub-acid fruit* (prunes are sweet fruits).

Pomegranate. Despite its tough skin and seed-filled pulp, the pomegranate contains nutrients beneficial to the body in excreting toxins. To eat this fruit, knead and squeeze it until soft. Then cut a small hole in the skin and suck out the pulp. The pomegranate may also be juiced. The juice blends well with carrot or apple juice. Class: *acid fruit*.

Potato: nightshade family. High in potassium, this starchy tuber is mainly an energy source. Bake lightly or cut and steam till tender. Class: *starchy vegetable*.

Pumpkin, marrow, and squash: gourd family. Including winter and summer squash and zucchini, this large variety of starchy, gourd family vegetables supply abundant potassium. Softer varieties like zucchini can be eaten raw; others must be steamed or baked. They provide essential nutrients used by the body in restoring health to the urinary and circulatory systems. Eaten raw, or hulled and roasted, pumpkin seeds are rich in nutrients needed by the body when restoring the prostate to healthy condition. All these vegetables are delicious when lightly baked with tomatoes and garlic. The traditional pumpkin pie should be made with only whole wheat flour, healthy oils, and unprocessed honey. Class: *starchy vegetable*.

Quinoa: goosefoot family. This native of the Andes may be the closest thing to complete protein found in the plant world. Available since 1984, quinoa is not a true grain but its calcium, B, and E vitamins and other essential nutrients are served as one. You can cook quinoa up alone, or use its gluten-free flour to make healthy breads and pastries. Class: *cereal*.

Radish: cruciferous family. Small, young radishes add zest to salads. (Large, older radishes become tough and fibrous.) Radishes are a healthful food only when not too pungent or "hot" to be eaten alone. They are mildly diuretic and their high fiber aids in preventing constipation. Class: *green vegetable*.

Raspberry: roe family. These small red, black, or purple berries grow wild in many northern areas and at higher elevations elsewhere. They provide nutrients utilized by the body in restoring carbohydrate metabolism. Class: *sub-acid fruit*.

Rhubarb: rhubarb family. Very lightly cooked rhubarb is a good source of calcium and potassium and aids in cleansing the lower intestines and bowels. Owing to its oxalic acid content, rhubarb should not be eaten too frequently if you're prone to kidney stones. Prepare it by placing cut rhubarb stalks in a pan of boiling water and removing immediately from the stove. Let stand a few minutes until ready. Do not allow rhubarb to become soft or mushy. Class: *green vegetable*.

Rice: grass family. Only unrefined brown or wild rice should be eaten. Organically grown long or short grain varieties are available inexpensively in most health food stores. Although rice is primarily a starch food, it is a good source of several B-vitamins and its high fiber speeds digestion and cleanses the bowels. This makes it very desirable in arthritis reversal. Prepare rice in a pressure cooker or simmer in a crockpot. Mix one cup of rice with 2 cups of water until boiling. Then cover and reduce heat for 35 minutes. Overcooking reduces its nutritional value. Far from boring, you can also eat rice as non-gluten rice flour, rice milk, amasake (a refreshing, sweet drink made from rice), and sweet, pounded rice called mochi. Other rice varieties include basmati, wehani, texmati, and sweet rice. Class: *cereal*.

Rutabaga: cruciferous family. Often called a Swedish turnip, this starchy root vegetable is a good source of calcium and calories. Steam briefly mixed with potatoes and other vegetables. Class: *starchy vegetable*.

Rye: grass family. Cooked cracked or whole, rye forms a good breakfast cereal, or it can be eaten with vegetables. Rye flour is also used in baking. Class: *cereal*.

Salmon. Rich in omega-3 oils and deliciously sweet, salmon is the king of fish. Serve this delicacy hot or cold, or try one of the several varieties such as chinook, sockeye, coho, or pink salmon to enjoy its arthritis benefiting qualities. Class: *protein*.

Sardines: True sardines are found mainly in Mediterranean waters. In the U.S. and Canada, most of these fatty, high protein, and calcium fish are canned. Our fresh domestic sardines are actually immature herring and anchovies, good foods in their own right. Class: *protein*.

Sesame seeds: pedalium family. Rich in calcium, minerals, and protein, sesame seeds rank with sunflower seeds as one of the most nutritious and healthful foods. Sesame seeds mix well with sunflower seeds in a ratio of about four parts sunflower seeds to one part sesame seeds. An oily butter called tahini is made from sesame seeds and, when fresh, is a fine, health-building food. Likewise, fresh, cold-pressed sesame seed oil is suitable for cooking. Class: *protein*.

Shiitake mushroom: yeast family. The shiitake, or Japanese forest, mushroom has a mild smoky flavor that makes soups more tempting; it's lentinan and vitamins make it a worthy addition to your arthritis program. If you're lucky and find fresh shiitake mushrooms in your local market, pick fragrant ones with firm flesh and caps that are still slightly closed. Dried shiitakes, sold in health food and grocery stores, must be soaked three to four hours before using. Discard the stems, then add both caps and soaking water to whatever dish you're preparing. Class: *neutral vegetable*.

Soybeans: (see Beans)

Spinach: goosefoot family. The several varieties of this green leafy vegetable supply a number of key nutrients needed by the body for arthritis recovery. Spinach is best chopped and added to salads, or it may be very briefly cooked. Most people overcook spinach, thereby releasing its oxalic acid which tends to bind calcium. Class: *green vegetable*.

Strawberry: rose family. Like the cherry, the strawberry has proved beneficial in helping the body heal itself from arthritis. Class: *acid fruit*.

Sunflower seeds: aster family. So rich are sunflower seeds in protein, calcium, iron, and vitamins A, E, and B-complex that many nutritionists consider them almost essential for bodily healing. Eat them alone or with sesame seeds and flavor with raisins. They can also be eaten with citrus fruits or with vegetable salads. Freshly-prepared sunflower seed oil, butter, and flour retain many of the key nutrients found in the seeds. Class: *protein*.

Sweet potato: morning glory family. Primarily an energy source, the sweet potato and yam also contain an abundance of vitamins, minerals, and beta-carotene. They are best baked in their jackets but may also be steamed, grilled, or casseroled. Class: *starchy vegetable*.

Tomato: nightshade family. The tomato plays a key role in supplying the body with nutrients used in healing. Tomatoes are best picked when ripe as commercial tomatoes are picked green and never achieve the flavor or juice content of homegrown ones. Tomatoes combine well with protein or green vegetables and are best eaten raw in salads or in sandwiches. They can also be stewed, broiled, baked, or made into soup. Class: *acid fruit*.

Trout (rainbow): salmon family. This beautiful fish is best eaten fresh out of the stream. It retains some of the healing fatty acids so beneficial in arthritis. Class: *protein*.

Tuna (albacore): mackerel family. The fine, white flesh of tuna is delicious when served fresh. While lower in fat than other fish, it's highest in protein at 25 percent per 100 grams[103]. Class: *protein*.

Turkey: turkey family. Light-colored turkey meat yields ten times as much whole protein as fat and is also a good source of phosphorus and potassium. Class: *protein*.

Turnip: cruciferous family. Both white and yellow varieties may be grated and eaten raw, or they can be lightly steamed, baked, or used in soup. Turnip greens are valuable sources of vitamin C and calcium and other nutrients required by the body in restoring health. Class: *starchy vegetable*.

Walnuts: walnut family. The several varieties including butternut and black walnuts are all good sources of protein, calcium, phosphorus, potassium, and omega-3 fats. Walnuts supply the body with nutrients utilized in reducing inflammation. Class: *protein*.

Watercress: mustard family. This crisp, peppery-tasting leafy vegetable is rich in vitamins and calcium and supplies a variety of nutrients essential to the body's healing powers. Add it to salads or use in sandwiches along with cucumber, tomatoes, and alfalfa sprouts as a bitter digestive aid. Class: *green vegetable*.

Wheat: grass family. Cooked cracked wheat or wheat berries make an enjoyable breakfast cereal while whole grain wheat flour may be used for baking. While bleached or refined wheat flour, including any products made from white flour, is totally devitalized; whole wheat is a good source of fiber, iron, phosphorus, and B-vitamins. Class: *cereal*.

Yeast: yeast family. One tablespoon of brewer's yeast supplies 3.9 grams of protein, 21 grams of calcium, 175 mgs. of potassium, 23 mgs. of magnesium, 1.7 grams of iron, and several B-complex vitamins. Unless you are allergic to it, brewer's yeast is a fine health-building food. Class: *protein*.

Yogurt, non or lowfat: bovid family. One cup of low-fat yogurt supplies the following percentages of U.S. recommended daily allowance: whole protein 30 percent; riboflavin 30 percent; calcium 40 percent; vitamin B_{12} 20 percent; and phosphorus 35 percent. Low in fat but high in energy, low fat yogurt supplies many essential nutrients required for bodily healing and friendly bacteria for the gut. Eat it alone, with bread, or with salads or other foods. Class: *protein*.

Zapote: plum family. The brown, black, yellow, and white varieties of zapote are fruits of Mexico and are all high in nutrients required by the body in reversing arthritis. Several varieties are grown in South Florida. The black zapote is filled with a soft, dark flesh that resembles cream and can be eaten with a spoon. It can be used as a creamy dressing on fruit salads. All zapotes, in fact, can be blended and used as cream or as desserts. Class: *sweet fruit*.

Appendix B

Drugs That Steal

Nutrients

Many medications, including those you take to ease arthritic suffering, play havoc with vitamins and minerals. They may decrease their absorption, increase excretion by the body or interfere with effective nutrient utilization by cells.

And like everything involving human beings, these drug-nutrient interplays are not simple. Your health, quality of your diet, age, and how long you've been taking these drugs all make a difference. People who have been sick for a long time, just had surgery, or have recently overcome an infection need more vitamins and minerals. If you've got digestive problems, or your liver isn't in tip-top shape, then your nutrient troubles caused by drugs magnify. Even when you take medicines—with or without meals—impacts how vitamins will be affected.

Here's a short list of how and what arthritis medications are affecting your nutrient status.

Drug	Nutrient Affected	How
Acetominophen	Vitamin C	Very high doses of this vitamin can inhibit acetominophen excretion thus causing potential toxicity.
Allopurinol	Iron	This drug impairs iron absorption.

Aspirin	Iron	Aspirin can cause gastrointestinal bleeding. Blood loss can cause iron deficiency.
	Folic acid	Aspirin increases folic acid loss through the urine.
	Vitamin C	Aspirin depletes the body's reserve of vitamin C. Twelve or more aspirin can cause deficiency signs like bleeding gums and bruising.
	Vitamin B_1	Aspirin increases excretion of this vitamin.
	Vitamin K	Less likely than other nutrients, nevertheless aspirin may decrease vitamin K levels.
Colchicine	All nutrients	This anti-gout medicine can cause malabsorption of all vitamins and minerals by destroying sections of your intestinal lining where food-digesting enzymes are found. Diarrhea can also be a problem, which increases loss of potassium, calcium, and magnesium.
Corticosteroids	Calcium	This anti-inflammatory drug pulls calcium from bones and decreases absorption of this mineral.
	Potassium	Corticosteroids enhance potassium loss from the body.

	Zinc	Zinc excretion increases while taking this drug.
	Vitamin B_6	Body reactions that use B_6 accelerate when steroids are taken, thus need for this vitamin increases.
	Vitamin C	Like B_6, vitamin C dependent reactions speed up as well as an increase in excretion. Both of these drug responses may create a vitamin C deficiency.
Cyclophosphamide	Sodium	This drug increases sodium loss.
Indomethacin	Iron	This drug causes microscopic bleeding in the gut, and thus iron deficiency through blood loss.
Methotrexate	All nutrients	This drug damages your gut lining, thus impairs overall nutrient absorption.
Sulfasalazine	Folic Acid	This drug decreases absorption of folic acid[104, 105, 106].

Appendix *C*

Looking for a Natural

Health Practitioner

There is a wide variety of natural health practitioners available to help you, from herbalists to naturopathic physicians. Practitioners' education is also diverse ranging from self-taught to doctoral degrees in their field. As a wise consumer it's up to you to ask lots of questions about a practitioner's training, years of practice, and knowledge and experience with arthritis.

Here's some questions you should ask.

1. Ask for referrals from friends and professional organizations (see listing below). Make sure you talk to several people before choosing your caregiver to get a clear, objective view of a practitioner's skills.

2. Ask your potential practitioner how he usually treats arthritis. Make sure these treatments are ones you feel comfortable with.

3. Does your practitioner treat every person with arthritis the same? If so, this is a red flag. An experienced practitioner recognizes that each individual has different needs, and responds differently to treatment.

4. Does the practitioner promise a cure? Another red flag. There is no guarantee a therapy will work until you try it. There are no perfect treatments ideal for everyone, as everyone responds in a different way to various therapies.

5. Have an open, honest discussion with the practitioner about your needs and wants, and his attitudes. Be suspicious if a caregiver doesn't want to talk with you beforehand. Remember you are paying him for a service.

6. Pick a practitioner who's willing to work along side any other doctor you choose to hire, including rheumatologists and MDs who practice more conventional medicine. The more practitioners work together for the good of the patient, the quicker you, the patient, will heal. Integrating the best of both natural and conventional medical care is the wave of the future.

7. Even if you have a good idea of who you want for a practitioner, interview others as a comparison.

If there's no one in your area, consider hooking up with a doctor who conducts telephone consultations; many of the below associations can help you out. While practicing medicine long distance is far from ideal, for those without local natural health care resources it's the second best thing.

During your search for a "Phone Practitioner," keep the above questions in mind. Especially important is number six. Find a conventional physician in your area who's open-minded and willing to discuss new ideas with you. Be frank with your local doctor about working with a natural consultant, and that you'd like him to share your medical records and treatments with your phone practitioner.

In the Doctor's Office

You've found the perfect doctor, now you can relax. Maybe not. The more proactive you are as a patient, the quicker you'll heal and the better treatment you'll receive. Use these pointers as a guide.

Ask Questions

When your physician examines you, ask about his or her findings and what they mean. Ask why lab tests are ordered and what the results indicate. If you're uncomfortable about the choice of treatment, press for an explanation. If you've read about another therapy you'd like to try, share that information with your doctor. Anytime you feel your doctor has missed something or hasn't asked pertinent questions, say so. Remember, you know your body better than anyone—including your doctor.

Change Doctors

Your doctor provides you with a service, and you should be comfortable with him or her. If you are uneasy with your choice of physician, consider looking for another. A large part of healing is the rapport between you and your health care provider.

Obtain Copies of Medical Records and Laboratory Reports

Ask for copies of your medical notes, as well as X-rays, blood tests, and other procedures. It's useful to maintain an at-home accurate file on your health for future medical visits. You can save valuable time by collecting medical records, and you'll be more knowledgeable about your medical history.

Learn About Your Condition

Educating yourself about the symptoms as well as conventional and alternative treatments available for your type of arthritis equips you with the tools to ask your doctor relevant questions. This will also help you decide when and if you need a second opinion.

Natural Health Database

Below is a comprehensive roster of various organizations that can help you find a natural health practitioner in your area. We've listed several types of caregivers so you have a choice.

The United States

American Association of Acupuncture and Oriental Medicine
433 Front Street
Capasauqua, PA 18032
PHONE: 610-433-2448
FAX: 610-264-2768

Referral lists of licensed acupuncturists and practitioners of Oriental Medicine are available for a donation fee. General information on these treatments are also available.

American Association of Naturopathic Physicians
2366 Eastlake Avenue East, Suite 322
Seattle, Washington 98102
PHONE: 206-323-7610
FAX: 206-323-7612

This professional organization also provides referrals to naturopathic physicians in your area. Literature on naturopathic medicine is also available.

American Chiropractic Association
1701 Clarendon Boulevard
Arlington, Virginia 22209
PHONE: 703-276-8800
FAX: 703-243-2593

The ACA will make referrals to a chiropractor in your area. They are also a wealth of information on chiropractic treatments.

American Herbalists Guild
PO Box 1683
Soquel, California 95073
PHONE: 408-469-4372
FAX: 408-469-4140

The AHG will refer you to a professional herbalist in your region at no cost. For a small fee, educational materials and reading lists regarding herbs, and their practicing herbal membership directory are also available.

American Holistic Medical Association
4101 Lake Boone Trail, Suite 201
Raleigh, North Carolina 27607
PHONE: 919-787-5181
FAX: 919-787-4916

The AHMA has a directory of holistic MDs and osteopathic doctors, naturopathic, and chiropractic physicians. They can direct you to one specializing in arthritis in your area.

The Raj (Maharishi Ayur-Veda Clinic)
1734 Jasmine Avenue
Fairfield, Iowa 52556
PHONE: 800-248-9050
FAX: 515-472-2496

The Raj is an Ayurvedic health clinic that can give you the name of a doctor in your area who practices Maharishi Ayur-Veda (one type of ayurvedic medicine). If there is no one near you, phone consultations are available from an experienced doctor for a fee. Free educational materials are also available.

National Center for Homeopathy
801 North Fairfax, Suite 306
Alexandria, Virginia 22314
PHONE: 703-548-7790
FAX: 703-548-7792

The mission of the NCH is to promote health through homeopathy. For a small fee, this organization will provide you with an information packet which includes professional homeopaths around the U.S. and Canada. Consumers are welcome to join.

The Rheumatoid Disease Foundation
5106 Old Harding Road
Franklin, Tennessee 37064
PHONE/FAX: 615-646-1030

This non-profit foundation furnishes referral lists of physicians (MDs, naturopathic physicians, osteopathic doctors, and chiropractors) who use natural therapies to treat arthritis. They are also a warehouse of information on various alternative arthritis treatments.

Canada

Maharishi Ayur-Veda College
500 Wilbrod Street
Ottawa, Ontario
Canada KIN 6N2
PHONE: 613-565-2030
FAX: 613-565-6546

This college also has a listing of Canadian ayuruedic practitioners. If you wish more information on this system of treatment, request to be placed on their mailing list.

Canadian Naturopathic Association
4174 Dundas Street, Suite 304
Etobicoke, Ontario
Canada M8X 1X3
PHONE: 416-233-1043
FAX: 416-233-2924

This professional group offers referrals to naturopathic doctors throughout Canada.

References

1. Eisenberg, D. M. et al. Unconventional medicine in the United States. *The New England Journal of Medicine* 1993; 328:246–52.

2. "Arthritis Foundation warns of future epidemic: CDC issues new report on arthritis prevalence" (press release), *News from the Arthritis Foundation* (Atlanta, GA), June 23, 1994.

3. "Diet & Arthritis Fact Sheet." Arthritis Foundation, Atlanta, GA.

4. "Rheumatoid Arthritis" Arthritis Information pamphlet, page 19. Arthritis Foundation, Atlanta, GA.

5. Darlington, L. G. and N. W. Ramsey. Diets for rheumatoid arthritis (letter). *The Lancet* 1991, November 9;338:1209.

6. Newman, N. M. and R. S. M. Ling. Acetabular bone destruction related to non-steroidal anti-inflammatory drugs. *The Lancet* 1985; ii:11–13.

7. Dunkin, M. A. and M. O'Koon. "The Drug Guide," *Arthritis Today*, July–August 1995, pp. 29–42.

8. Quick Takes, *Arthritis Today*, October 1995.

9. Kelley, W. N. et al. (eds.). *Textbook of Rheumatology*, (4th ed.), *vol.* 2. Philadelphia: W. B. Saunders Company, 1993.

10. Following Doctor's Orders. *Arthritis Today*, July–August 1995, pp. 16.

11. Faulkner, G. et al. Aspirin and bleeding peptic ulcers in the elderly. *British Medical Journal* 1988; 297:1311–1313.

12. Orange, L. M. The high cost of managing NSAID-induced ulcers. *Family Practice News* 1993; 23(1):16.

13. Mordechai, R. et al. Hepatotoxicity of nonsteroidal antiinflammatory drugs. *The American Journal of Gastroenterology* 1992; 87(12):1696–1704.

14. Poole, Judith. Too much emphasis on drugs. *Arthritis Today,* January–February 1996, pp. 6–7.

15. Potera, Carol. Prednisone use in RA. *Arthritis Today,* March–April 1995, pg. 8.

16. Anon. Gold therapy in rheumatoid arthritis (editorial). *The Lancet* 1991; 338:19–20.

17. Morgan, Brian L. G. *The Food & Drug Interaction Guide.* New York: Simon & Schuster, 1986.

18. Arthritis Foundation. "Arthritis Facts" information sheet, 1995.

19. Benjamin, C. M. et al. Joint and limb symptoms in children after immunisation with measles, mumps, and rubella vaccine. *British Medical Journal* 1991; 304:1075–1078.

20. Mitchell, L. A. et al. Chronic rubella vaccine-associated arthropathy. *Archives of Internal Medicine* 1993; 153: 2268–74.

21. Sanchez-Guerrero, J. et al. Postmenopausal estrogen therapy and the risk for developing systemic lupus erythematous. *Annals of Internal Medicine* 1995; 122:430–433.

22. Orange, L. M. Group of GPs failed to diagnose Lyme disease presenting as arthritis. *Family Practice News* 1993; 23(1):16.

23. Schumacher, H. R. et al. (eds.). *Primer on the Rheumatic Diseases* (10th ed.). Atlanta: Arthritis Foundation, 1993, pp. 118.

24. Tierney, L. M. et al. (eds.). *Current Medical Diagnosis & Treatment* (35th ed. 1996). Stamford: Appleton & Lange, 1996, pg. 725.

25. Donovan, P. "Osteoarthritis," Seattle, WA (unpublished paper and personal communication).

26. Star, V. L. Gout: options for its therapy and prevention. *Hospital Medicine* 1995, November:25–28.

27. Anon. "You are what you eat . . .". *Food & Water Journal*, Winter 1996; 5(1):5.

28. van de Laar, M. A. F. J. and J. K. van der Korst. Rheumatoid arthritis, food, and allergy. Seminars in Arthritis and Rheumatism 1991; 21(1):12–23.

29. Inman, R. D. Antigens, the gastrointestinal tract, and arthritis. *Nutrition and Rheumatic Diseases* 1991; 17(2):309–321.

30. Pizzorno, J. and M. Murray. *A Textbook of Natural Medicine*. Seattle: John Bastyr College Publications, 1987.

31. Eaton, K. K. et al. Gut permeability measured by polyethylene glycol absorption in abnormal gut fermentation as compared with food intolerance. *Journal of the Royal Society of Medicine* 1995; 88:63–66.

32. Nordlee, J. A. et al. Identification of a brazil-nut allergen in transgenic soybeans. *The New England Journal of Medicine* 1996; 334:688–692.

33. Pizzorno, J. and M. Murray. *A Textbook of Natural Medicine*. Seattle: John Bastyr College Publications, 1987, III: Fasting.

34. Sundquist, T. et al. Influence of fasting on intestinal permeability and disease activity in patients with rheumatoid arthritis shows normalization during fasting. *Scandinavian Journal of Rheumatology* 1982; 11:33–38.

35. Pizzorno, J. and M. Murray. *A Textbook of Natural Medicine*. Seattle: John Bastyr College Publications, 1987, IV: Bw/Tox, pp. 5, 6.

36. Pizzorno, J. and M. Murray. *A Textbook of Natural Medicine*. Seattle: John Bastyr College Publications, 1987, IV: WestDi, pg. 2.

37. Russell, Robert. Nutrition and Aging/Gastrointestinal Tract. Nutrition Action Health Letter. May 1992; 120(5):825–828.

38. Brostoff, J. and S. T. Challacombe. *Food Allergy and Intolerance*, Philadelphia: Bailliere Tindall, 1987.

39. Darlington, L. G. and N. W. Ramsey. Diets for rheumatoid arthritis. *The Lancet* 1991; 338:1209.

40. The Burton Goldberg Group. *Alternative Medicine: The Definitive Guide*. Puyallup: Future Medicine Publishing, Inc., 1993, pg. 47.

41. Patterson, R. (ed.). *Allergic Diseases: Diagnosis and Management (4th ed)*. Philadelphia: J. B. Lippincott, 1993, pg. 364.

42. U.S. Department of Health and Human Services. *The Surgeon General's Report on Nutrition and Health*. Rocklin: Prima Publishing, 1988.

43. Literature from Oldways Preservation and Exchange Trust, Cambridge, MA.

44. Sacks, F. M. and W. W. Willett. More on chewing the fat. The good fat and the good cholesterol. *The New England Journal of Medicine* 1991; 325(24):1740–42.

45. Lichenstein, A. H. Trans fatty acids and hydrogenated fat—what do we know? *Nutrition Today* 1995; 30(3):102–107.

46. Callegari, P. E. and R. B. Zurier. Botanical lipids: potential role in modulation of immunologic responses and inflammatory reactions. *Nutrition and Rheumatic Diseases* 1991; 17(2):415-425.

47. Geusens, P. et al. Long-term effect of omega-3 fatty acid supplementation in active rheumatoid arthritis. *Arthritis & Rheumatism* 1994; 37(6):824–829.

48. Pizzorno, J. and M. Murray. *A Textbook of Natural Medicine*. Seattle: John Bastyr College Publications, 1987, VI: Gout.

49. "Diet in principle: Basic for nutrition competence." Handout from University Health Clinic, Seattle, WA.

50. Harman, D. Aging: prospects for further increases in the functional life span. Age 1994; 17:119–146.

51. Longevity: can science extend the human lifespan?: *The University of Texas Lifetime Health Letter* 1993, September; 5(9):1 & 6.

52. Murray, M. and J. Pizzorno. *Encyclopedia of Natural Medicine.* Rocklin: Prima Publishing, 1991.

53. Bunker, V. W. The role of nutrition in osteoporosis. *British Journal of Biomedical Science* 1994; 51(3):228–40.

54. Zeng, Q. et al. Osteoarthritis: clinical and epidemiological investigation (Chinese). *Chung-Hua Nei Ko Tsa Chih Chinese Journal of Internal Medicine* 1995; 34(2):88–90.

55. Nelson, M. E. et al. A one-year walking program and increased dietary calcium in postmenopausal women: effects on bone. *American Journal of Clinical Nutrition* 1991; 53:1304–11.

56. Situnayake, R. D. et al. Chain breaking antioxidant status in rheumatoid arthritis: clinical and laboratory correlates. *Annals of the Rheumatic Diseases* 1991; 50(2):81–6.

57. Anon. Ames agrees with Mom's advice: eat your fruits and vegetables. *The Journal of the American Medical Association* 1995; 273(14):1077–78.

58. Shils, M. E. and V. R. Young. *Modern Nutrition in Health and Disease (7th ed.).* Philadelphia: Lea & Febiger, 1988, pg. 53.

59. Weiss, R. F. *Herbal Medicine.* England: Beaconsfield Publishers, Ltd., 1991, pg. 258.

60. Hoffman, D. *The Holistic Herbal.* Scotland: Findhorn Press, 1986, pg. 132.

61. Kennedy, A. R. The evidence for soybean products as cancer preventive agents. *Journal of Nutrition* 1995; 125(3 Suppl.):733S–743S.

62. Gao, B. Y. et al. Effect of panaxatriol saponins isolated from Panax notoginseng (PTS) on myocardial ischemic arrythmia in mice and rats (Chinese). *Acta Pharmaceutica Sinica* 1992; 27(9):641–4.

63. Koyama, N. et al. Inhibitory effect of ginsenosides on migration of arterial smooth muscle cells. *American Journal of Chinese Medicine* 1992;20(2):167–73.

64. Liu, Y. P. et al. Protective effects of fulvotementosides on acetaminophen-induced hepatotoxicity. *Acta Pharmacologica Sinica* 1992; 13(3):209–12.

65. Bartram, H. P. et al. Does yogurt enriched with Bifidobacterium longum effect colonic microbiology and fecal metabolites in healthy subjects? *American Journal of Clinical Nutrition* 1994; 59:428–32.

66. Losacco, T. et al. Immune evaluations in cancer patients after colorectal resection (Italian). Giornale di Chirurgia 1994; 15(10):429–32.

67. Bhutta, Z. A. et al. Dietary management of persistent diarrhea: comparison of a traditional rice-lentil based diet with soy formula. *Pediatrics* 1991; 88(5):1010–1018.

68. Johnson Schulte, M. Yogurt helps to control wound odor (letter). *Oncology Nursing Forum* 1993; 20(8):1262.

69. McNutt, K. R. The individualized prescriptive foods era has dawned. *Nutrition Today* 1993, May/June:43–47.

70. Anon. Fish oil and the development of atherosclerosis. *Nutrition Reviews* 1987; 45(3):9091.

71. Kremer, J. M. et al. Effects of high-dose fish oil on rheumatoid arthritis after stopping nonsteroidal anti-inflammatory drugs. *Arthritis & Rheumatism* 1995; 38(8):1107–1114.

72. Carper, Jean. *The Food Pharmacy*. New York: Bantam Books, 1988, pp. 191, 193, 321.

73. Personal communication. Donovan, Patrick, ND, Seattle, WA.

74. Ziboh, V. A. et al. Effects of dietary supplementation of fish oil on neutrophil and epidermal fatty acids. *Archives of Dermatology* 1986; 122:1277–82.

75. Stenson, W. F. et al. Dietary supplementation with fish oil in ulcerative colitis. *Annals of Internal Medicine* 1992; 116:609–614.

76. Stammers, T. et al. Fish oil in osteoarthritis. *The Lancet* 1989; 11(8661):503.

77. Carroll, K. K. Biological effects of fish oils in relation to chronic diseases. *Lipids* 1986; 21:731–32.

78. Rudin, D. O. and C. Felx. *The Omega-3 Phenomenon*. New York: Rawson Associates, 1987, pp. 23, 125.

79. Murray, M. *The Healing Power of Herbs*. Rocklin: Prima Publishing, 1995, pp. 70, 327.

80. Srivastava, K. C. and T. Mustafa. Ginger (Zingiber officinale) in rheumatism and musculoskeletal disorders. Medical Hypotheses 1992; 39:342–348.

81. Pizzorno, J. and M. Murray. A *Textbook of Natural Medicine*. Seattle: John Bastyr College Publications, 1987, VI: Gout; V: Curcum.

82. Blazso, G. and M. Gabor. Anti-inflammatory effects of cherry (Prunus avium L.) stalk extract. Pharmazie 1994; 49:540–541.

83. Lauerman, J. F. Asian herbal therapy for lupus. *Alternative & Complementary Therapies* 1996; 2(1):16–18.

84. Henricksson, A. E. K. et al. Small intestinal bacterial over-growth in patients with rheumatoid arthritis. *Annals of the Rheumatic Diseases* 1993; 52:503–510.

85. Tassman, G. C. A double-blind crossover study of a plant protelolytic enzyme in oral surgery. *Journal of Dental Medicine* 1956; 20(2):51–53.

86. Journal of Ethnopharmacology, 1988, volume 22.

87. Pizzorno, J. and M. Murray. A *Textbook of Natural Medicine*. Seattle: John Bastyr College Publications, 1987, V: Bromel.

88. Personal communication and correspondence. Ilene Dahl, ND, LAc, Concord, CA.

89. Serdula, M. K. et al. Fruit and vegetable intake among adults in 16 states: results of a brief telephone survey. *American Journal of Public Health* 1995; 85(2):236–239.

90. Heliovaara, M. et al. Serum antioxidants and risk of rheumatoid arthritis. *Annals of the Rheumatic Diseases* 1994; 53:51–53.

91. Goldenberg, D. L. Fibromyalgia, chronic fatigue syndrome, and myofascial pain syndrome. *Current Opinion in Rheumatology* 1995; 7(2):127–135.

92. Kelley, W. N. et al. *Textbook of Rheumatology* (*vol. 1* (*4th ed.*). Philadelphia: W. B. Saunders Co., 1993, pg. 471.

93. Veale, D. et al. Primary fibromyalgia and the irritable bowel syndrome: different expressions of a common pathogenetic process. *British Journal of Rheumatology* 1991:30(3):220–222.

94. Hedges, H. H. The elimination diet as a diagnostic tool. *American Family Practice Journal* 1992; 46(5):77S.

95. Hostmark, A. T. et al. Reduced plasma fibrinogen, serum peroxides, lipids, and apolipoproteins after a 3-week vegetarian diet. *Plant Foods for Human Nutrition* 1993; 43(1):55–61.

96. Goldman, S. I. et al. Phenobarbital-induced fibromyalgia as the cause of bilateral shoulder pain. *Journal of the American Osteopathic Association* 1995; 95(8):487–490.

97. Romano, T. J. Exacerbation of soft tissue rheumatism by excess vitamin A: case reviews with clinical vignette. *West Virginia Medical Journal* 1995; 91(4):147.

98. Anon. Is fibromyalgia caused by a glycolysis impairment? *Nutrition Reviews* 1994; 52(7):248–250.

99. van Vollenhoven, R. F. et al. Dehydroepiandrosterone in systemic lupus erythematosus. *Arthritis & Rheumatism* 1995; 38(12):1826–1831.

100. Hall, G. M. et al. Depressed levels of dehydroepiandrosterone sulphate in postmenopausal women with rheumatoid arthritis but no relation with axial bone density. *Annals of the Rheumatic Diseases* 1993; 52(3):211–214.

101. Anon. Estrogen may alleviate carpal tunnel syndromes. *Medical World News* 1992; 17.

102. Eisinger, J. et al. Selenium and magnesium status in fibromyalgia. *Magnesium Research* 1994; 7(3–4):285–288.

103. Wood, R. *The Whole Foods Encyclopedia*. New York: Prentice Hall, 1988.

104. Lewis, C. W. et al. Drug-nutrient interactions in three long-term-care facilities. *Journal of the American Dietetic Association* 1995; 95:309–315.

105. Trovato, A. et al. Drug-nutrient interactions. *American Family Practice* 1991; 44:1651–1658.

106. Morgan, B. L. G. *The Food & Drug Interaction Guide.* New York: Simon & Schuster, 1986.

Index

Arthritis, (*Continued*)
  tendonitis, 36
  vitamin deficiency, 49
  wheat as worst food aggravator,
    135–36
Arthritis The Basic Facts, 12, 17, 23
Arthritis Foundation, 1–2, 12, 13, 16, 23,
  31, 54, 239
Arthritis Today, 12, 13, 239
Aspartame, 183
Aspirin, 8, 11–13, 50, 80, 306
  and food tolerance, 111
  and gout, 44
  and prostaglandins, 173
Atherosclerosis, 231
Attitude, 6
Autoimmunity, 4, 37, 56–59
  ankylosing spondylitis, 38 (*See also*
    Ankylosing)
  cross reactivity, 56
  dermatomyositis, 40
  gout, 42–44 (*See also* Gout)
  Polyarteritis Nodosa, 40
  Raynaud's Phenomenon, 39–40
  rheumatic fever, 40
  rheumatoid arthritis, 37–38
  scleroderma, 39–40
  Sjögren's Syndrome, 37–38
  systemic lupus erythematosus (SLE),
    29, 38–39
Ayurvedic medical system, 182, 243

Bacteria, non-toxic, 105–6
  growth of, encouraging, 232–33
Baker's Farmer's cheese, 206
Baker's yeast, 137
  testing of, 126
Barton-Wright, Dr. C.E., 230
Bartram, Hans-Peter, 233
Bellew, Dr. Bernard, 232
Beverages, restorative, 213–14
Bingham, Dr. Robert, 217, 231–32, 235,
  244
Bitters as recovery food, 250
Blackstrap molasses, 183
Blair, Dr. Ludwig N., 246
Blood circulation, improving, 231

Bowel problems, 52–53
  elimination, improving, 225–26
  healing, 97–98 (*See also* Digestive diet
    plan)
Bran not needed, 198, 259
Brewer's yeast, 137
  testing of, 126
Bromelain, 248
  in pineapple, 252
Brostoff, Jonathan, 110
Brown rice as recovery food, 254–56
Burkitt, Dr. Dennis, 226
Bursitis, 36
Butyric acid, 104

Caffeine as stressor in food, 114
  prohibited, 181
Calcium, 219, 221–22
  deficiencies, 49
Callegari, Dr. Peter, 172
Capsaicin, 239
Carbohydrates, 174–75
  complex, 209–10
  refined, as stressor foods, 114, 163
Carrot-apple-seaweed snack as recovery
  food, 247–48
Cartilage, 257
Cayce, Edgar, 170
Cayenne pepper as recovery food,
  239–40
  for fibromyalgia, 283
Celiac Disease, 136
Cereal as recovery food, 241–43
Challacombe, Stephen, 110
Chamomile as recovery food, 250
  tea, 101, 214
Chapattis, 126
Chemical additives prohibited, 181–82
Cherries as recovery food, 246–47
Chewing, greater need for, 102, 273
Chinese Medicine view of recovery
  foods, 253–54
Chlorophyll, 206–7
Cholesterol, 168–69
Cholinesterase, 137
Chronic atrophic gastritis, 53
Chronic fatigue syndrome, 280